Katiba BEROUAL

A natural pharmacy

Katiba BEROUAL

A natural pharmacy

Effect of flax on integument disorders

ScienciaScripts

Imprint

Any brand names and product names mentioned in this book are subject to trademark, brand or patent protection and are trademarks or registered trademarks of their respective holders. The use of brand names, product names, common names, trade names, product descriptions etc. even without a particular marking in this work is in no way to be construed to mean that such names may be regarded as unrestricted in respect of trademark and brand protection legislation and could thus be used by anyone.

Cover image: www.ingimage.com

This book is a translation from the original published under ISBN 978-620-3-43763-8.

Publisher:
Sciencia Scripts
is a trademark of
Dodo Books Indian Ocean Ltd. and OmniScriptum S.R.L publishing group

120 High Road, East Finchley, London, N2 9ED, United Kingdom
Str. Armeneasca 28/1, office 1, Chisinau MD-2012, Republic of Moldova, Europe
Printed at: see last page
ISBN: 978-620-6-01255-9

Contents

GENERAL INTRODUCTION

By intuition and experimentation, humans have selected food plants for nourishment, medicinal plants for healing, and poisonous plants for use as arrow poisons in hunting or warfare. [e] Despite a certain eclipse due to the rise of synthetic chemistry from the 19th century onwards, plant-based medicines are still widely used, both in developing and industrialised countries, where they are mainly used for self-medication (Lehmman, 2013).

The importance of phytotherapy is continuously increasing. Many patients prefer herbal medicines because of their good tolerance and low side effects.

Herbal medicines are approached much more scientifically. Indeed, research and evaluation methods for traditional medicine are based on the safety and efficacy of traditional herbal medicines and therapies (Patil et al, 2010). According to WHO (2000) guidelines, pre-clinical and clinical trials of these products are very similar to those for conventional medicines. In addition, the search for new active ingredients by pharmaceutical and academic laboratories has helped to explain and even approve some traditional uses (Guedje et al, 2012).

Over the years, several researchers have investigated different phytoconstituents and nutraceutical formulations with healing effects (Kumar et al, 2007; Sandhya et al, 2011; Shivhare et al, 2014a). Another aspect as important as the first one is represented by hair beauty products which constitute a significant part of the global cosmetic market. Hundreds of products for hair growth and maintenance are prepared by combining one or more herbal medicines (Ali and Ansari, 1997).

In addition, research into new feedstuffs is constantly being carried out to improve animal performance while limiting the adverse effects of feeding on animal health (Audureau, 2007).

Flax, among other things, is widely used in everyday public health and is also widely used in animal nutrition. It is not a new food; it is one of the oldest and perhaps one of the most original and precious foods because of its healing properties which have made it an age-old plant with medicinal virtues. Moreover, its Latin name "*Linum usitatissimum*" (flax of all uses) is well deserved (Weill and mairesse, 2010). Curiously, its oil is known for its softening and emollient properties. It protects and softens irritated skin. Moreover, flax (seed and oil) improves animal health and fertility parameters, while the answer to the question of zootechnical performance remains perplexing.

In Algeria, this plant is very little studied. The main objective of this study is to know the pharmaco-toxicological properties of this blue flower.

Our work contributes to a better understanding of the therapeutic value of *L. usitatissimum* through preclinical trials. Firstly, by exploring the impact of topical application of its oil on the healing process in experimental burns. Secondly, the effects of the oil and the seed on the hair system (hair growth and regrowth) are quantitatively evaluated. Finally, the safety of the prolonged ingestion of the seed and its impact on some zootechnical performances in rabbits are assessed.

The mode of presentation of this thesis is common, starting with a bibliographical part where are developed reminders on the structure and physiology of the skin and its appendices, the scarring process (especially during burns), alopecia, the place of phytotherapy in skin and hair disorders as well as a detailed overview on the importance of *Linum usitatissimum* in food and in therapy. The experimental part is devoted in a first chapter to the action of linseed oil on epithelial regeneration, and in a second chapter to the estimation of the effect of linseed (oral and topical test) on hair growth in rabbits. The safety is tested and confirmed by biochemical analyses, anatomopathological examinations of the emunctory organs, in the third chapter, and in the last chapter, an appreciation of the zootechnical performance of rabbits whose food ration is supplemented with ground flaxseed.

BIBLIOGRAPHY

CHAPTER I :
TEGUMENTARY SYSTEM

1. Skin

The skin, the second largest organ in the body after the skeleton, is of paramount importance for the vital survival of mammals (Chuong et al, 2002). The structure of the skin is derived from the embryonic ectoderm and mesoderm, which give rise to the epidermis and dermis, respectively (Hardy, 1992). Within these generalised layers of the tegument specialised structures are also derived from the ectoderm and/or mesoderm, including sensory nerves, sweat glands and hair follicles (Chuong et al, 2001).

1.1. Description

The skin is a tegument that covers the entire body. In the average adult its surface area varies between 1.2 and 2.2 m^2 ; it weighs 7% of the total body mass in humans (Schaffer and Mednche, 2004; Marieb, 2005). In which the thickness of the skin varies considerably from area to area to suit its specific functions, in general, the skin is thickest on the back and neck, and thinnest on the abdomen, sternum and in the axillary and inguinal regions (Monteiro et al, 1993; Noli, 1999).

It varies between 0.4 mm and 2 mm in cats, between 0.5 and 5 mm in dogs, between 1.7 and 6.3 mm in horses and 1.5 to 4 mm in humans (Silvetti, 1981; Guilbaud et al, 1993; Muller et al, 2001; Lapante, 2002; Tomczak , 2010).

The skin is an organ in its own right and is an indicator of general health, playing several fundamental roles (Malnoux, 1991; Viguier and Degorce, 1992; Scott et al, 1995; Wheater et al, 1995; Palazzi, 2002; Pavletic, 2003; Noli, 2006):

- Anatomical-physiological interface and protective barrier.
- Semi-permeable membrane (perspiration and absorption).
- The most extensive sensory organ in the body.
- Organ of organic synthesis and metabolic excretion.
- Production of vitamin D.
- Production of hair and pigmentation.
- Responsible for thermo- and immuno-regulation.
- Reserve of electrolytes, water, vitamins, fats and proteins.

1.2. Histology

The skin is made up of four regions (Figure 1) which are from surface to depth: the outer epidermis derived from the ectoderm and its appendages; the basement membrane or dermal-epidermal junction, the deeper dermis derived from the mesoderm; and the hypodermis or subcutaneous tissue, which corresponds to the superficial layer of the deep fatty tissue (Kierszenbaum, 2002). This hypodermis extends below the dermis and connects the skin to the underlying organs (Dadoune et al, 2007).

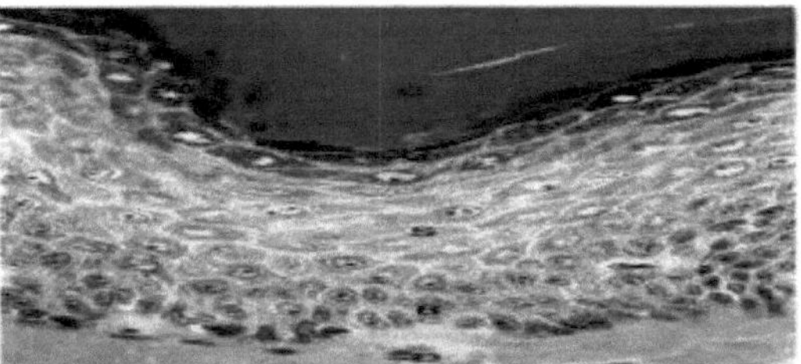

Figure 1: Various cell layers making up the epidermis (wheater et al, 1995) Dermis **(D)**, basal layer or stratum basal **(B)**, spinous layer or stratum spinosum **(S)**, granular layer or stratum granulosum **(G)** and horny layer or stratum corneum **(C)**.

1.3. Skin Appendages

In addition to the skin, the tegumentary system includes several subsidiary productions derived from the epidermis, with specific functions. These appendages reinforce the protective role of the skin. These are the hair and hair follicles, the nails, the sweat glands and the sebaceous glands. Each plays an important role in maintaining the body's homeostasis.

1.3.1. The pilosebaceous follicles

They are appendages of the skin (originating from the embryonic epidermis, but mainly located in the dermis and hypodermis (Prost squarcioni, 2006). They include the hair and its sheaths, sebaceous glands and, in some areas, an arrector muscle and/or apocrine sweat glands.

1.3.2. Sebaceous glands

They are exocrine glands (simple/complex) tubulo alveolar a

These are the holocrine secretion cells, often associated with hair follicles. Their secretory portion, located in the dermis, produces sebum which is made up of lipids.

It keeps the skin elastic by forming a film on the surface that covers the stratum corneum; in addition to this physical barrier role, sebum also forms a chemical barrier against pathogens. It also provides waterproofing of the coat and contains pheromones (Scott et al, 1995; Hillyer and Quesenberry, 1997). They are absent in hairless areas (Tomczak, 2010).

1.3.3. The sweat glands

They are of two types: eccrine glands independent of the hair and apocrine glands attached to the hair follicle. The former are present all over the skin surface, more numerous on the palms of the hands and soles of the feet, and produce sweat (Kohler, 2011). The latter, with apocrine secretion, are tubulo-contained exocrine glands (epitrichiales/ atrichiales) present in the armpits (axillae), perineum, external auditory canal and eyelids (Muller et al, 2001; Noli, 2006; Prost-squarcioni, 2006).

1.3.4. **The** hair-retaining **muscle**

It is a smooth muscle stretched between the dermal-epidermal junction and the sub-isthmic region of the hair; it runs along the outer surface of the sebaceous gland. Its contraction causes horripilation or vertical hair (Prost-squarcioni ,2006) (figure 2).

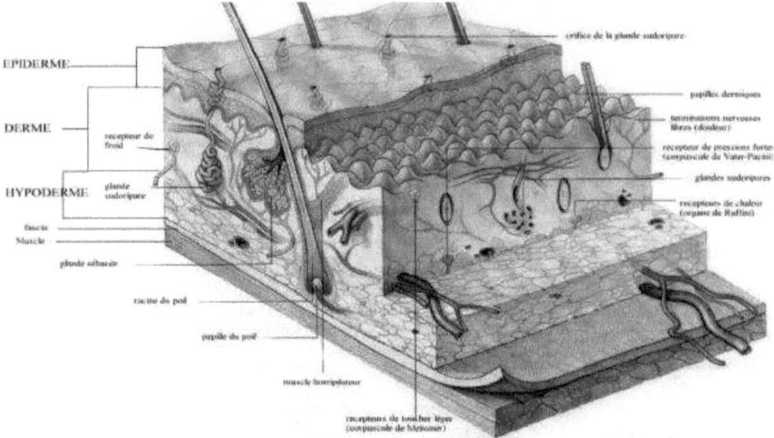

Figure 2: Scheme of the skin covering (Laplante 2002; Anonymous, 2011)

1.4. Claws and nails

They are specialised structures formed of continuously growing keratin produced by a complex ungual base. They are located at the digital extremities and have various roles (defence, grip, ambulation) (Bensegueni, 2007).

1.5. Blood vascularisation

Knowledge of the vascularisation of the skin is essential in the field of cutaneous reconstruction. The epidermis is not vascularised, like all epithelium, it is nourished by imbibition through the capillary networks of the dermal papillae, unlike the dermis and hypodermis, which are on the other hand richly vascularised by a highly systematised network of medium and small calibre arterioles, capillaries and venules. In the dermis, three interconnected blood vascular plexi exist (Figure 3). The most superficial is formed by small, loop-shaped capillaries which link the ascending arterioles and post-capillary venules. It provides nutrients to the epidermis and the infundibulum of the hair follicles. The middle plexus is located at the level of the sebaceous glands. It provides blood supply to the glands, erector muscles and follicular isthmus. The deep plexus, located under the hair follicles, at the fascia-hypodermis junction, supplies the dermal papilla, the apocrine glands and the other two plexi (Boutonnat, 2008; Ferraq, 2007; Lefort, 2011). In other words, according to Pavletic (1985), Bourges-Abella (2008), the vascularisation of the skin is characteristic; it includes a segmental vascularisation, a perforating vascularisation and a cutaneous or dermo-epidermal vascularisation.

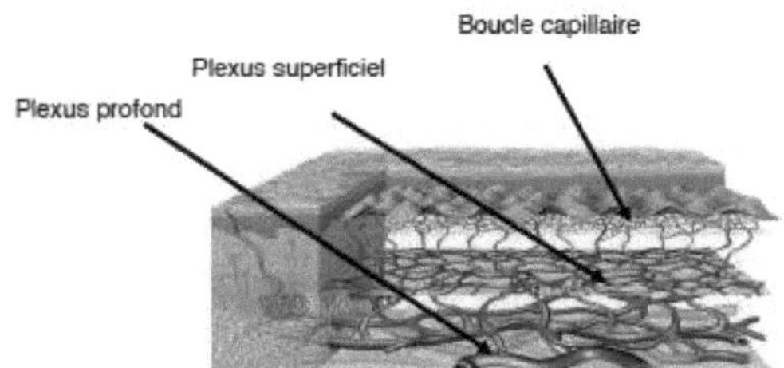

Figure 3: Vascularisation of the skin (Leonhardt, 2001)

1.6. Lymphatic vascularisation

Recalling that lymphatic vascularisation is parallel to that of the blood. Thus, the lymphatic plexus exists in the deep superficial dermis, whose distribution is very uneven throughout the body (Boutonnat, 2008; Anonymous, 2011). Also the transudate is transported by lymphatic vessels that originate in the capillary network of the superficial part of the dermis through a blind loop at the top of the dermal papillae and follow the path of the venous network (Viguier and Degorce, 1992). and the lymphatic capillaries originate from vessels originating from lymph nodes (Boutonnat, 2008; Anonymous, 2011).

1.7. Innervation

The nerves of the skin are sensory receptors and motor nerves, most of which innervate the epidermis and dermis, and are of somatic origin. All of them derive from spinal nerves, the endings of which perceive heat, cold, pressure, pain and pruritus, the information of which varies according to the intensity of the stimulus (Bensegueni, 2007).

1.8. Particularities of the skin in rabbits

According to the study of Oznurlu and his team (2009), the general skin characteristics of angora and New Zealand white rabbits were quite similar and showed a thin skin. The angora rabbit skin was significantly (p<0.05) thicker than that of the New Zealand white rabbit and the main difference was in the papillary layer of the dermis. The angora rabbit had the highest number of hair follicles in the dermis unit area. Due to typical tip examinations, the histological characteristics of the skin of the New Zealand white rabbit were suitable for the leather industry, while that of the angora rabbit had good hair follicle characteristics for wool production.

2. Hair

Hair plays several important functions in humans and mammals in general (Ebling, 1987). Several abnormalities can affect hair such as hirsutism and alopecia (Marieb, 1993).

Hair follicles are important reservoirs of stem cells that can regenerate the epidermis. They probably play an important role in wound healing (Morasso and Tomic, 2005). Thus, the quality of wound healing is affected in people with destroyed hair follicles.

2.1. Constitution

Hair is a filiform production of the epidermis. It partially or completely covers the skin of mammals. The hair is constituted from the inside to the outside: a medulla which contains air, glycogen vacuoles or pigments, a cortex composed of corneal cells and a cuticle whose role is protection by the characteristic assembly of its corneocytes (anucleated epithelial cells) (Thebault, 1977; Monteiro et al, 1993; Gentz et al, 1995; Scott et al, 1995)

The bulbar matrix overlying the dermal papilla that feeds it is the site of production of actively multiplying hair cells, which give rise to a particularly strong, fibrous-like keratin of low lipid content and high sulphide content, it is composed of "polypeptide chains. "Alpha helix" is the descriptive term given to the polypeptide chain that forms the keratin protein in human hair (Patil et al, 2010; Kohler, 2011).

The matrix allows the hair to acquire its pigmentation. It is protected by two sheaths: an inner epithelial sheath produced by the matrix that disappears at the isthmus of the hair follicle and an outer fibrous epithelial sheath (stem, hair bulb, dermal papilla) (Kohler, 2011).

2.2. Varieties

Depending on the amount of hair and sebaceous glands and the area where they terminate, three types of follicles can be distinguished: 'terminal', 'hairy or lanuginous' and 'sebaceous' (Sperling, 1991; Goodman and Gilman, 1996; Anonymous, 2011)

In rabbits, there are several types of hair: the visible silky hair is the guard hair, the down is shorter, finer and softer hair that is hidden under the guard hair (Arvy and More, 1975). At the section, the rabbit hairs are shaped like an eight (8) (Robert, 1982).

The vibrissae are prominent, mechanoreceptors involved in tactile sensitivity (Arvy and More, 1975; Mcewan and Jenkinson, 1970; Breathnach and Bannister, 1995).

2.3. Functions

In humans, the main function of hair is to smell insects before they bite. Hair protects the head from injury and has a cosmetic function. They prevent heat loss and protect from the sun. Nose hairs filter out large dust particles and insects from the inhaled air (Ferraq, 2007).

In animals, the coat acts as a thermal insulator and a protective barrier against mechanical aggression and the sun's ultraviolet rays. It also allows the animal to be camouflaged in its environment, to be recognised socially by its coat (Courtin-donas, 2009) and is involved in visual and olfactory communication via pheromones (Alhaidari and Von tscharner, 1997).

2.4. Growth

In humans, the average hair growth phase is 30-45 days. He loses about 100/100,000 hairs per day. The average life span of a hair is 4.5 years. The hair falls out and is replaced within 6 months by a new hair follicle which undergoes an activity cycle. (Patil et al, 2010) The hair growth cycle consists of three phases: anagen (period of active growth), catagen (period of breakdown and change) and telogen (end of the resting period before growth resumes) (Soma et al, 1998; Oznurlu et al, 2009).

2.5. Moulting process

According to Sandford (1979) and Lebas et al (1996), there are two moults depending on the age of the rabbit: the juvenile: newborn, infant, sub-adult coat and the seasonal: spring and autumn. Factors involved in moulting also affect coat quality: photoperiodism, temperature, hormones (thyroid) and inadequate nutrition (pathology and poor hygiene).

The synchronisation of the hair cycle is lost after the second wave of moult shortly after birth. Hair moults independently and seasonally, which is not seen in humans (Chuong et al, 2001; McElwee and Sinclair, 2008).

3. Hair follicle
3.1. Definition

The hair follicle *(folliculus* = small sac) in mammals is an invagination of ectodermal origin; like the epidermis with which it is continuous, it sinks more or less deeply into the dermis depending on the size of the hair it produces (Olivera-Martinez et al, 2004).

3.2. Classification

Hair follicles are classified into primary and secondary follicles. Primary follicles are large in diameter and are deeply rooted in the dermis and are usually associated with sebaceous and sweat glands. Secondary follicles are smaller in diameter. Their roots are superficial and may have a sebaceous gland. They do not have a sweat gland or an arrector muscle. (Monteiro-Riviere, 1998).

Many differences exist in the arrangement of hair follicles in animal species (Alhaidari and Von Tscharner, 1997; Monteiro-Riviere, 1998; Moore et al, 1998). Thus, they are either located individually, in single follicles, or located in compound follicles, in one or clusters of several hair follicles located in the dermis and which usually contain a primary hair follicle and several secondary follicles (Alhaidari and Von Tscharner, 1997; Monteiro-Riviere, 1998; Broeck et al, 2001).

3.3. Structure

The hair follicle is made up of individualised compartments. Some are of dermal origin (connective sheath and dermal papilla), others of epithelial nature (external epithelial sheath, internal epithelial sheath, hair shaft and sebaceous gland) (Marieb, 1993; Commo and Bernard, 1997; Thibaut et al, 2005; Gagnon, 2005). The hair also has appendages: a sebaceous gland, the whole forming the pilosebaceous unit and the arrector muscle (Marieb, 1993).

Figure 4 shows a longitudinal section of the pilosebaceous unit of the follicle which is divided into several compartments: the infundibulum, the superficial portion above the sebaceous gland duct. Continuous with the interfollicular epidermis, the isthmus, which is a short portion between the duct of the sebaceous gland and the protuberance of the arrector muscle, the bulge where the latter is attached and finally the lower segment ending in the hair bulb (Geras, 1990).

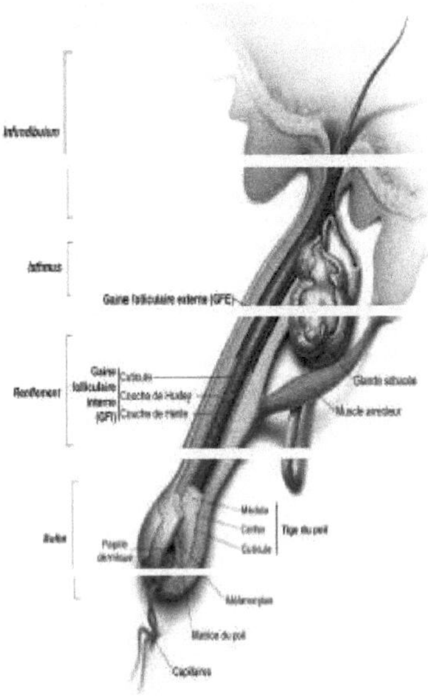

Figure 4: Pilo-sebaceous unit (Gagnon, 2005)

3.4. Hair cycle

The hair follicle goes through several growth cycles during which each hair undergoes 3 successive phases. A growth phase, anagen phase (I-VI), a catagen phase, resting phase and a telogen phase (Fuchs et al, 2001; Yu et al, 2006; Peterschmitt, 2009).

The duration of each phase depends on the type and location of the hair follicle (Vogt et al, 2008).

3.4.1. Anagenic phase

This is the growth phase of the hair (divided into 6 stages) during which it grows continuously. It is characterised by rapid proliferation of follicular keratinocytes, elongation and thickening of the hair shaft (Paus and Cotsarelis, 1999) and intense mitotic activity in the vascularised bulb. The root of the old hair is pushed to the surface as the new hair grows and emerges from the old hair follicle (Stenn and Paus, 2001).

The work of Thebault (1977) confirms that the rate of growth is specific for each category, in rabbits it increases rapidly until 6-7 weeks after hair removal and becomes specific between the 9th and 13th week. In humans, the duration of the anagen phase of the healthy scalp hair follicle, the main determinant of its length, is usually two to six years (Paus and Cotsarelis, 1999).

3.4.2. Catagen phase

The active growth phase is followed by a transition phase which lasts about two weeks. During these two phases, mitoses come to an abrupt halt, the regression phase, during which the lower two thirds of the hair enter into programmed cell death (apoptosis), characterised by a cessation of protein and pigment production, involution of the follicle and a fundamental restructuring of the extra matrix. This leads to regression and shortening of the hair (Fuchs et al, 2001; Stenn and Paus, 2001).

3.4.3. Telogen phase

The hair follicle regresses to less than half its size in the anagen phase. The resting phase is also called the quiescence phase. It lasts about 3 months (Stenn and Paus, 2001). Morphologically, all that remains is a peg of epithelial cells overlying a cluster of resting papillae skin cells (Fuchs et al, 2001). The shortening resulting from the regression of an epithelial strand is associated with an upward displacement of the dermal papilla within the connective tissue sheath of the follicle. The hair shaft evolves into a cluster of hairs, which is held tightly in the bulbous base of the follicular epithelium, before it is discarded from the follicle, most often as a result of combing or washing.

It is not resolved or confirmed whether the excretion of telogen hair (teloptosis) is also an active regulated process or a passive event that occurs at the beginning of the anagen sequence (Paus and Cotsarelis, 1999; Pierard-Franchimont and Pierard, 2001).

3.4.4. Kenogenic phase

After the resting phase, the matrix reactivates and forms a new hair that will replace the fallen hair or delodge it if it is still present (Fuchs et al, 2001). The hair follicle is empty after shedding of the hair fibre, but before the onset of new hair growth, it is at a stage called "kenogen" which can be observed in healthy skin. However, the frequency and duration of these stages are significantly higher in people with androgenetic alopecia (Rebora and Guarrera, 2002).

3.5. Cycle control

Season, nutrition, age, sex, health and hormonal status of the animal are factors that affect the hair growth cycle (Paus et al, 1990; Lanszki et al, 2001).

-Cytokines, hormones, neuropeptides and pharmaceuticals are growth factors influencing cyclical changes (Paus, 1998; Paus and Cotsarelis, 1999). Indeed, the relative duration of phases varies with hormonal factors (Moretti et al, 1976). Other physiological factors, pathological factors, location, age and nutritional status affect the phases (Randall et al, 1991; Randall et al, 1992; Kang-Bong et al, 2011).

-In addition, when hair is induced in the anagen phase, there is an increase in the activity of the enzymes, Y-glutamyl transpeptidase (Y-GT) and alkaline phosphatase (ALP), which are indicators of hair growth (Hattori and Ogawa, 1983).

-Hormone Growth Insulin-like growth factor-I (GH-IGF-I) may have functions in the maintenance of human skin integrity.

It is involved in promoting hair growth by regulating cell proliferation and migration during hair follicle development (Paus and Cotsarelis, 1999). It is possible that IGF-I, produced by the skin cells of the papilla, may act on keratinocytes, stimulating the proliferation of these keratinocytes in hair follicles. Studies have shown the importance of IGF-I in maintaining the morphology of normal skin (Hattori and Ogawa, 1983) and in increasing collagen synthesis by fibroblasts *in vitro* (Harrison et al, 2006), thereby increasing skin elasticity (Harada and Okajima, 2007; Harada et al, 2008).

-Stress induced hair growth inhibition is promoted by the nerve growth factor (NGF), (Peters et al, 2004). Several studies have shown that stress has negative effects on the hair follicle (Rupniak and Kramer, 1999; Hadshiew et al, 2004).

3.6. Hair characteristics in rabbits

The different breeds of rabbit differ in the nature and colour of the hair and in the size of the animal (Djago et al, 2010). This is related to the longer duration and speed of hair follicle activity which allows the hair to grow for more than 14 weeks. This difference is explained by the presence of a recessive gene carried by the Angora rabbit (Sandford, 1979; Lebas et al, 1996; Allain, 2007).

Although the study by Allain (2007) suggested that the unusual length of Angora hair is a result of the longer growth period and increased growth rate, the results show that the matrix of hair follicle germ cells of the Angora rabbit had a higher rate of protein synthesis in addition to the mitotic index compared to the New Zealand White rabbit. These results provide histo-morphological evidence for comparisons between the performance traits of the two strains. This confirms the presence of strain-specific characteristics and inter-breed variations in skin layer thickness and number of follicles in a rabbit skin surface unit (Oznurlu et al, 2009).

CHAPTER II:
TEGUMENT DISORDERS

1. Burns

Numerous traumas of multiple origins frequently cause significant tissue lesions, by their mechanical action, they give wounds and provoke a solution of continuity of the tissues by their physical action; burns which are wounds without solution of continuity but with tissue lesions which can go from the simple erythema to the carbonization. These lesions must be treated in order to create the necessary conditions for a rapid and correct evolution of the scarring process, which is a complex phenomenon passing through different phases that follow one another before leading to a definitive scar within a few months. This allows the restoration and optimal recovery of the functional integrity of the skin (Bensegueni, 2007).

1.1. Definition

Burns are a serious danger to the skin, as they cause destruction of the skin covering and sometimes even the underlying structures (Diouri et al, 2003, Dif et al, 2010).

Burns are defined as either physical trauma to the skin and mucous membranes, or tissue damage or necrosis.

They lead to protein clotting, heavy exudation and the development of infections (Fayolle, 1992; Swaim and Henderson, 1997). On the surface of destroyed cells, ooze is observed; this protein and electrolyte containing body fluid causes dehydration and electrolyte imbalance.

This in turn leads to renal failure and hypovolemic shock (Mitz, 1994; Marieb, 2008), which can have a major impact on the whole body (physical and/or psychological) (Le Bever, 2009).

1.2. Etiology and severity

The causes of burns are infinite but can be classified into four main groups: thermal, electrical, chemical and radiological. In all cases, there is destruction of the skin, but we can oppose the burns where this destruction is fast and massive (thermal and electrical burns), to the one where it is slower, over several hours (chemical burns) or several days.

In the first case, the initial clinical picture is dominated by a shock proportional to the mass of the injured tissue, in the second case the appearance of lesions is torpid (Bargues and Carsin, 2003). According to Guilbaud et al (1993) and Zinai (2008), the severity of a burn is conditioned by many parameters:

- Nature of the vulnerable agent and duration of exposure
- Type of accident (domestic, work)

- Time to treatment
- Quality of the means used
- Extent, depth and location of lesions
- Impairment of vital functions (upper airways)
- Impairment of the function of the areas concerned
- Age and background of the victim

Assessing the severity of a burn is difficult and requires considerable clinical experience. Assessing the severity of a burn means knowing the area affected, the depth of the damage and its location (Bargues and Carsin, 2003).

1.3. Area reached (extent)

It determines the prognosis and the nature of the treatment (Probst, 1984; Swaim et al, 1990; Swaim et al, 1996) and can be estimated by measuring the weighted area, dividing it by the total body surface area and multiplying the result by 100. In an emergency, this assessment meets the Wallace "rule of nine" (Moisson, 1998). For small areas, the burns should be redrawn on a diagram and the area calculated from the tables of Lund and Browder (Descamps et al, 2011).

1.4. Depth

Burns are classified according to their depth into three or even four categories: first degree, second degree (superficial and intermediate), and third degree (Figure 5). They correspond to a histological classification based on the damage to the regenerative basement membrane of the epidermis (Fayolle, 1992; Farstved and Stashak, 2008).

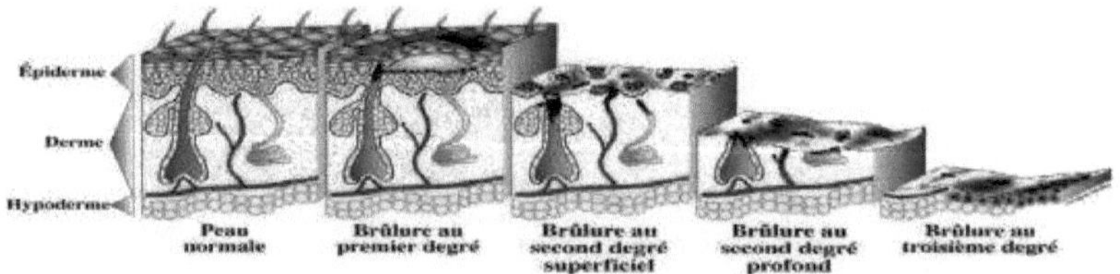

Figure 5: Diagram of the different degrees of skin burn (Marieb, 1993)

1.5. Location

It must be taken into consideration because it modulates the prognosis, in fact, scarring reactions can have a severe impact on functional recovery (Bensegueni, 2007).

The location has two dangerous lesions, namely vital and functional. The first is accompanied by a significant reddening of the face and neck and an infectious risk in the perineum. The second is in the hands and feet, where the deep, circular lesions form a tourniquet that does not allow for expansion of the redness but creates vascular compression (Bargues and Carsin, 2003).

1.6. Pathological anatomy

According to Djenane (1997), the burned area consists of three zones of tissue reaction, which are related to the depth of injury (degree of burns): A central zone, which has had the greatest contact with the heat source. It is characterised by necrosis and is called a coagulation zone.

At the periphery of this is the zone of capillary stasis. It is marked by tissue and vascular lesions which are reversible.

The zone of hyperthermia is similar to a superficial burn. It is characteristic of the inflammatory response (vasodilation of the microcirculation, synthesis of prostaglandin E2) (Jonston, 1993)

Under the action of different factors, such as oxygen pressure, hypovolemia, infection, microvascular lesions may appear and deepen the initial lesion; on the first day, a deep 2nd degree lesion may transform and become a 3rd degree lesion on the third day (Fayolle, 1992; Echinard and Laterjet, 1993).

1.7. Pathophysiology

The destruction of burnt skin leads to two types of consequences: Consequences related to the destruction of cells, resulting in capillary, osmotic and cellular disorders.

Consequences related to the suppression of its own functions, which develop through sensitisation to infection and metabolic disorders with disturbances of thermoregulation (Guilbaud et al, 1993).

The severity of injury depends on the temperature and time of exposure, the traumatic agent; glowing object, hot liquids, hot gases as well as the structure of the tegument, glabrous skin or presence of dander (hair or feathers); cell death starts from 40°C for a six hour exposure (Williams, 1999).

The lesion caused by the burn provokes an inflammatory reaction that affects the body. This reaction evolves in two stages, firstly a pro-inflammatory phase (characterised by a systemic response inflammatory syndrome) followed by an anti-inflammatory phase marked mainly by immunosuppression. These inflammatory phenomena have important pathophysiological consequences, particularly on circulatory homeostasis and endothelial integrity, to the point where they are capable of threatening the vital prognosis. The inflammatory reaction can be amplified or maintained by intercurrent events, such as infection; capable of inducing veritable vicious circles that perpetuate the initial reaction (Ravat et al, 2011).

1.8. Pain

The burn is an external aggression par excellence, which comes to devastate a life, gives a particular intensity to the word "pain".

It is obvious that the pain of the burn victim must be treated for humanitarian reasons, but also and above all because painful phenomena can be a serious obstacle to the healing of the resulting burn (Joucdar, 1993).

Given the complexity and multiplicity of mechanisms involved in pain, the importance of initiating effective analgesic therapy quickly and adjusting it according to the changing needs of patients must be emphasised. (Choiniere, 2000).

1.9. Treatment

Traumatology is a frequent and important pathological aspect of human and veterinary medicine that practitioners must deal with in an effort to treat successfully.

Wounds and burns are traumas of the skin and mucous membranes whose frequency and severity have justified research to improve their therapeutic management. Depending on the severity of the burn, treatment is either by application of anti-inflammatory drugs, excision of necrotic tissue, use of artificial epithelium, or mucosal transplantation, grafting and reconstruction (Latarjet et al, 1992).

Local treatment is one of the components of the overall treatment of burns. Its role is fundamental since it is the skin lesions which not only cause and maintain the general disease, but also cause the sequelae. Local treatment aims to restore tegumental integrity, either by healing superficial lesions or by reconstruction in the case of deep lesions. It includes specific procedures to achieve healing and to prepare the lesions before surgery, during which the surfaces concerned are disinfected and treated with anti-infectious or non-infectious topicals (hydrogel, hydro colloids) and excisions and coverings of the excised areas (Branswyck, 2009).

Autologous skin grafts are still the basic technique for treating deep burns, but it needs to be adapted when the burns are extended by expanding skin samples or supplemented by the use of other methods, such as skin allografts, autologous keratinocyte cultures or artificial skin (Dhennin, 2002).

In a certain number of patients, secondary interventions will also be necessary, there are always sequelae which, whatever their location and extent, are very painful and which the initial local treatment should aim to limit (Dhennin, 2002).

The goal of burn reconstruction is to restore function, but also aesthetics to allow the trauma patient to be fully reintegrated into society (Costagliola, 2011).

Man has always used plants since ancient times to relieve many ailments. The healing activity of plants is recognised in all civilisations. This "natural pharmacy" has always been the subject of numerous scientific studies (Habbu et al, 2007; Kumar et al, 2007; Sandhya et al, 2011; Shivhare et al, 2014a). A part of chapter III is devoted to the synthesis of healing plants.

2. Healing

The skin is a very exposed organ. Skin destruction can be of various origins (traumatic, infectious, tumoral, vascular, iatrogenic). Its repair corresponds to healing. Depending on the surface and depth of the lesion, the closure of the skin covering will be spontaneous, obtained by local care (directed healing) or will require surgical treatment (Bruant-rodier, 2005).

2.1. Definition

It is the natural biological phenomenon of repairing localized lesions in human and animal tissues through the set of processes or phenomena of repair and regeneration (Grimbert, 2009). A distinction can be made between two basic wound healing processes: first and second intention (Coulibaly, 2008).

2.2. First intention

It occurs within a few days. When there is good contact between the edges of the wound, in the absence of a hematoma, and when emergency care has been carried out with perfect asepsis. In general, it results in a clean, linear scar which improves over the following six months (Fabre, 1982).

2.3. Second intention

It is a healing of the wound with loss of substance. It occurs whenever there is no reunion of the edges of the wound or when, due to a local complication, usually infectious, the wound has become disunited. Healing, whether it is first or second intention, theoretically takes place in three phases according to Fournier and Mordon, (2005) (figure 6).

- The vascular and inflammatory phase, with clot formation, recruitment of inflammatory cells (wound detersion).
- The tissue repair phase (epithelialization of the wound).
- The remodelling of the extracellular matrix and scar maturation.

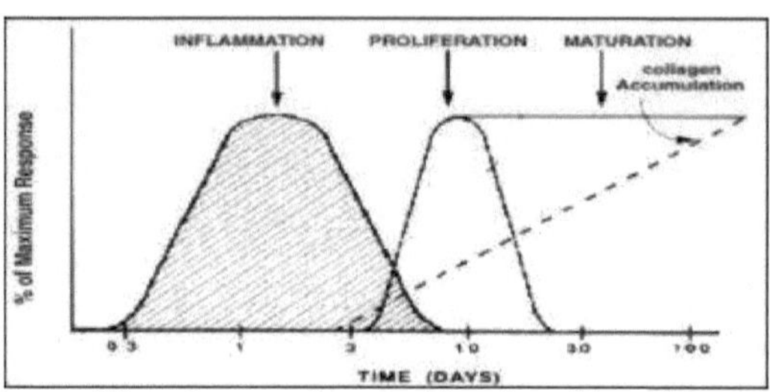

Figure 6: Chronology of the phases of wound healing (Fournier and Mordon, 2005)

2.3.1. Detersion phase

According to Borel and Maquart (1998), it corresponds to the elimination of all tissue residues and foreign bodies that would have the effect of preventing the connective tissue from budding. Its importance in time varies with the nature of the wound. "This phase begins approximately six (6) hours after the appearance of the wound by vasomotor reactions, resulting in the production of a liquid exudate at the wound level, rich in plasma proteins (histamine, phagocytin), lysosomal enzymes (proteinases, nuclease, phosphatase), ions (Na+ K+) and cellular elements (leucocytes: polynuclears, monocytes)

Polynuclear cells and monocytes migrate together to the wound. Polynuclear cells are the most numerous and have phagocytosis activity, they die quickly in three to five days. "Mononuclear cells are less numerous, but have a longer life span, and multiply greatly, with macrophagic activity" (Frekha, 1988).

2.3.2. Inflammatory phase

In this constructive phase, the phenomena aimed at filling the tissue gap can begin, through the reparative, fibroblastic and epithelialization phase.

- A repair phase

This phase corresponds to the development of the fleshy bud, which grows from the depths to fill the loss of substance. Thus, in the connective tissue at the periphery of the lesion, the indifferent mesenchymal cells are transformed into migrating fibroblasts, guided by the fibrin network which serves as a guiding thread, the fibroblasts travel in close association with blood and lymphatic neoformations and form the granulation tissue (Fabre, 1982)

- A fibroblastic phase

First of all, the fibroblasts elaborate:

- The elements of the fundamental substance are mainly mucopolysaccharides (responsible for the high water content of the granulation tissue) and glycoproteins with high antigenic power.

22

\-   The pro-collagen which is excited in the extracellular medium is transformed into tropocollagen under the influence of hydrolysis (Frekha, 1988), this tropocollagen in the organisation of a long double twisted helix, gives rise to collagen fibres.

At the end of this period, which lasts two to three weeks, the capillaries inflect in a plane perpendicular to their initial direction and anastomose with each other, the budding process comes to an end, it is responsible for filling the wound by its synthesis activity and for the contraction of this wound which leads to a reduction in its surface area, at which point the epithelialization stage begins (Fabre, 1982).

2.3.3. Epithelialization phase

The end result of this phase is wound coverage, epithelialization occurs concentrically from the wound edges, and over a period of time that varies greatly depending on the nature, location and extent of the wound.

The basal marginal cells enlarge, flatten and progress, which are driven by the expulsive force of adjacent cells, during mitosis. This progression takes place along the epidermal edge of the wound, and the mode of migration of the epidermal cells has been compared to a caterpillar-like movement, with the keratinocytes appearing to roll over each other.

When the wound is filled with granulation tissue, epithelial cell sliding occurs later and only ceases due to contact inhibition. The initial stimulus for wound healing, in particular epithelialisation, has not been clearly identified (Maurin, 2005).

According to Borel and Maquart (1998), this is either a positive stimulation due to wound hormones or a release of a control provided by a mitotic inhibitor called chalone.

All in all, healing is the result of phenomena of varying intensity depending on the extent and type of the aggression, the extent of the tissue damage that is articulated, in a more or less harmonious way.

In order to restore the initial tissue integrity, there are also individual factors, some of which are unknown and unpredictable, that are involved in the correct course of these phenomena (Verola, 2006).

When the phases of healing are proceeding normally, the colour code is visualised. At detersion, black means a necrotic wound, yellow a fibrinous wound, and green an infected wound. At budding, red can be found, pink of a healing reminds epithelialization (Duquennoy, 2009).

Under natural conditions, contraction is the main route to healing, and planimetric study allows direct quantitative assessment by calculating the wound area and its evolution over time and by assessing the quality of granulation tissue (Ono et al, 1999). Using the equation of Lodhi et al (2006) or Srivastava and Durgaprasad (2008), the percentage of wound contraction is obtained.

2.4. Other modes of healing

According to the bibliography cited by Tomczak (2010), there are other mechanisms of epithelial regeneration, namely: subcrustaceous, desiccation, 1ere delayed intention and 3eme intention.

2.5. Pathological development

According to Bruant-Rodier (2005), there are several scars, the hypertrophic and cheloidal ones, the hyperkeratotic ones, the dyschromic ones, and the unstable ones. Among the inesthetic (pathological) scars, a distinction must be made between those that are defective, linked to an error in the suturing technique, and those that are truly pathological involving the healing phenomena themselves (Andree Mathieux, 2011).

The synthesis of the pathological evolution of the scar of the two different natures (septic and aseptic) is illustrated in Table I.

Table I: Septic and aseptic scar evolution

Nature	Evolution	References
Septic	Wound infection	Tomczak, 2010
	Wound dehiscence	Asimus, 2001; Aguerre, 2004)
	Persistent suppurations	Foweler, 1993; Delverdier et al,
	hot abces and fistulas	1993
Aseptic	Vascular alteration :	
	Hemorrhages and hematoma	Deodhar and Rana 1997
	(Iderne	Remdios, 1999
	Ischemie	He, 2006
	Seromas: fluid collections.	Masonc et al, 1993; Pavletic, 2003
	Alteration of the	
	budding:	Waldron and Zimermman, 2003;
	Atonic wound	He, 2006
	Ulcers	He, 2006
	Inflammatory granuloma	He, 2006
	ChaoMe	Asimus, 2001
	. . . . .	
	Alteration of the epithelialization phase	
	Delayed epithelialization	Tomczak, 2010
	Entropion of the wound	He, 2006

3. Alopecia

Basically, any change and/or irregularity in the three biological factors of hair follicle density, namely: hair follicle dimensions, number of hairs per unit of skin surface and length of growth cycle, implies the acquisition of disorders and guides the diagnostic approach in an individual (alopecia or hypertrichosis) (Mcelwee and Sinclair, 2008). The impact of hair disturbance and hair loss on human life is harmless, but the impact on quality of life and emotional well-being is disproportionate to its dimensions.

3.1. Definition

Hair loss is the thinning of hair on the scalp. The medical term for it is alopecia. Alopecia can be temporary or permanent. The most common form of hair loss occurs gradually and is called "androgenetic alopecia", which means that a combination of hormones (androgens) and heredity (genetics) is required to develop the condition (Patil et al, 2010).

3.2. Frequency and cause

Androgenetic alopecia (AGA), also called male pattern hair loss or male pattern baldness in men and female pattern hair loss in women, affects at least 50% of men by age 50, and up to 70% of all men in later life (Norwood, 1975).

Estimates of its prevalence in women have varied widely, according to data from Reygagne (2009), 10% of women develop diffuse hair loss from the age of 20, 30% from the age of 40 and 45% after menopause; although other studies state that six per cent of women under the age of 50 are affected, it is increasing to a proportion of 3040% of women aged 70 years and over (Norwood, 2001)

The incidence of androgenetic alopecia is more common in Caucasians than in Black or Asian individuals. Among Caucasians, the percentage of men with baldness increases with age worldwide: 25% at 25 years, 30% at 30 years and older, 40% at 40 years, 50% at 50 years (Roy et al, 2008; Clere, 2010). The age of onset is variable. In fact, androgenic alopecia can start as early as puberty. The earlier it occurs, the greater the risk of it being significant (Clere, 2010).

Some scientists consider testosterone to be one of the main causes of hair loss. Testosterone is closely related to heredity.

Another point of view is the insufficient and/or unbalanced nutrition of the blood flow. Hair loss in men and women is also caused by excess oil in the scalp. These three factors are the most common causes of hair loss.

These include: emotional sources, stress and nervous disorders, ageing, infections, hormonal imbalance, polluted environment, toxic substances, injuries and radiation (Roy et al, 2008).

3.3. Pathophysiology

Androgenic alopecia (AGA) is hereditary and androgen-dependent, clinically defined by progressive thinning of the hair or miniaturisation of the follicle. While the genetic involvement is pronounced but poorly understood, significant progress has been made in understanding the key elements of androgen metabolism involved.

The androgen-dependent process is primarily due to the binding of dihydrotestosterone (DHT) to the androgen receptor (AR). DHT-dependent cellular functions are related to the availability of weak androgens, their conversion to the more potent androgen by the action of 5alpha reductase, the low enzymatic activity of androgens (enzyme inactivation) and the functionally active nature of the ARs present in large numbers (Trueb, 2009).

Exposure of the scalp predisposed to high levels of DHT and increased expression of AR, as well as conversion of testosterone to DHT in the dermal papilla play a central role, while androgens (modulating factors) derived from the dermal papilla cells are likely to influence the growth of other hair follicle components. The result is a decrease in hair follicle size accompanied by a decrease in the duration of the anagen phase and an increase in the percentage of hair follicles in the telogen phase (Cotsarelis and Millar, 2001).

On histological examination of scalp biopsies, miniaturisation of terminal hairs is frequently associated with perifollicular lymphocytic infiltration and ultimately fibrosis (Jaworsky et al, 1992; Whiting, 1993).

Therefore, it is conceivable that the role of follicular inflammation, or microscopic fibrosis, has been underestimated, it seems likely that this is what would prevent the follicle from reforming into a terminal hair follicle (Trueb, 2002).

3.4. Other forms

Other types of hair loss include alopecia (patches of baldness that usually grow backwards), traction alopecia (thinning of tight braids or ponytails) and telogen effluvium (rapid hair loss after childbirth, a fever or sudden weight loss) (Patil et al, 2010)

3.4.1. Pelade (*Alopecia Areata*)

It is an unpredictable autoimmune disease that has a histopathologically variant feature at different stages and presents as non-scarring hair loss, although the exact pathogenesis of the disease remains to be clarified.

Prevalence rates of the disease of 0.1% to 0.2% have been estimated for the USA. *Alopecia Areata* (AA) can affect any area of hair. It often presents as limited areas of hair loss without scarring on normal-looking skin, so it is likely that the timing and severity of alopecia is determined by an interaction between a genetically predisposed individual and exposure to a triggering environmental factor.

The course of the disease is unpredictable and the response to treatment can be variable (Alkhalifah et al, 2010; Wang and Mcelwee, 2011).

3.4.2. Telogen effluvium (without alopecic plaque)

In this case, hair loss is most often acute or subacute and is the result of telogen conversion of the hair follicles followed by hair loss within 2 months. It is followed by normal regrowth.

There are many causes: *postpartum* alopecia, after a high fever, various infections, inflammatory diseases (lupus erythematosus) or surgical shock.

To a lesser degree, there is a seasonal physiological telogen effluvium in autumn and spring. It does not require any treatment, since it is followed by normal regrowth. Psychological care is essential, as this "hair loss" often has a major psychological impact. It is important to reassure patients that the symptoms are generally transient (Descamps et al, 2002).

3.4.3. Medicated alopecia

Hair loss secondary to medication is rare and poorly understood, except in the case of anti-cancer therapies. However, a number of drugs frequently dispensed in pharmacies are likely to cause alopecia. Alopecia remains an undesirable effect of anticancer chemotherapies because these substances act through a direct, toxic effect on the anagenic phase (Pillon, 2013).

The incidence (mean estimate 65%) and severity of chemotherapy-induced alopecia (CIA), is variable and related to the particular chemotherapeutic protocol. CIA is traditionally classified as acute diffuse hair loss caused by dystrophic anagen effluvium, which presents with different clinical types of hair loss (Trueb, 2009).

The other drugs that most frequently cause hair loss are psychotropic drugs and antihypertensive drugs, due to the inhibition of mitoses, secondary to the reduction in the production of cyclic adenosine monophosphate (cAMP), associated with the inhibition of the effects of catecholamines and responsible for the vasodilation of peripheral blood vessels. The secondary vasoconstriction would then favour capillary fall. Aldosterone antagonist diuretics act through an antiandrogenic effect. Conversion enzyme inhibitors (CEI) appear to cause reversible hair loss (enalapril, captopril). The use of these drugs, when associated with renal insufficiency, is thought to cause zinc deficiency, responsible for symptoms such as alopecia (Pillon, 2013).

3.5. Therapeutic modalities

3.5.1. Pharmaceutical molecule

The aim of the therapeutic challenge is to increase the coverage of hair on the scalp and to delay the progression of hair thinning.

Two drugs approved by the US Food and Drug Administration (FDA) are available for this purpose, oral finasteride, at a dose of 1 mg per day and topical minoxidil solution (Price, 1999).

- **Finasteride**

It is a competitive type II 5 a-reductase inhibitor and inhibits the conversion of testosterone to dihydrotestosterone (DHT). The rationale for using finasteride to treat androgenic alopecia (AGA) is based on the absence of alopecia due to congenital type II 5 a-reductase deficiency in men, and the presence of both 5a-reductase and DHT in the degenerated scalp (Kaufman et al, 1998).

Hair regrowth was observed in 48% of patients receiving finasteride for one year, it is generally well tolerated, but a few have withdrawn from the 'treatment programme' due to associated sexual dysfunction (Upadhyay *et al,* 2012a,b). Finasteride is contraindicated in women who are or may become pregnant (Trueb, 2002; McClellan et al, 1999) because 5a-reductase can cause external malformations of the genitals in male fetuses (Trueb, 2002).

- **Minoxidil**

It promotes hair growth by increasing the duration of the anagen (Buhl, 1989). It stimulates the resting hair follicle to grow (Trueb, 2002) by increasing the size of miniaturised hair follicles and enlarges suboptimal follicles in parallel with the initiation of anagen growth in telogen phase hair follicles (Sinclair, 1998; Otberg et al, 2007). While minoxidil was developed for the treatment of hypertension, and this feature of the drug's action is best understood, its mechanism of action on hair growth is somewhat poorly understood.

Minoxidil is a potassium channel opener and vasodilator and has been reported to stimulate VEGF production in cultured dermal papillae cells (Lachgar et al, 1998).

Topical solutions of 2-5% minoxidil are available for the treatment of AGA in men and women (Li et al, 2001).

Unfortunately, the efficacy of minoxidil is variable and temporary, which makes it difficult to predict the success of treatment on an individual basis. Restrogens and anti-androgens are used in women with AGA, although no studies have been conducted.

When a combination of a restrogen and a progestin is prescribed for contraception or hormone replacement therapy in women with AGA, care should be taken to choose a progestin that is androgen-free, or preferably has anti-androgenic activity, for example cyproterone acetate (Price, 1999; Trueb, 2002). The associated side effects of pruritus, dryness, scaling, local irritation and dermatitis should be reported (Spindler, 1988).

It is likely that several other molecular approaches to hair and follicle enlargement remain to be discovered.

The therapy of hair loss disorders interferes with aggravating stressors, therefore the comprehensive and careful management beyond the drug and prescription to alleviate patients' clinical symptoms are the concomitant psychological implications (Hadshiew et al, 2004).

3.5.2. Other modality

The main approach to minimising chemotherapy-induced alopecia is scalp cooling. Unfortunately, most published data on scalp cooling are unproven. Several experimental approaches to the development of pharmacological agents are being evaluated including drug-specific antibodies, hair growth modifiers, cytokine growth cycle factors, antioxidants, inhibitors of apoptosis and cell cycle and proliferation modifiers.

No specific pharmacological intervention is available to manage stress-induced hair loss in humans. An effective therapeutic intervention in this regard would have the effect of prolonging the anagen phase of the hair cycle, thus preventing the premature onset of catagen (Paus and Cotsarelis, 1999). The latter is indicated in "rebellious" alopecia (Clere, 2010).

CHAPTER III:
NATURAL PRODUCTS

1. New substances

There is a widespread belief that natural health products (NHPs) are safe and less toxic than pharmaceuticals. This may explain their popularity for the maintenance of general health as well as their use against various problems such as dermatological ones (Millar, 1997). Indeed, the importance of phytotherapy is increasing. Many patients prefer herbal medicines because of their good tolerance and low side effects. In addition, herbal medicines are approached much more scientifically (Eichele, 2010). With the advancement of biology and biological chemistry as well as the generalisation of the use of natural substances as therapeutic agents, the target must necessarily possess a potential activity or be related to biological processes. It can be observed that each isolation of a natural product (innovation carrier) is necessarily accompanied by biological tests (Corbu, 2008).

The term "safety pharmacology studies" first appeared in the International Conference on Harmonisation of Technical Requirements for the Registration of Pharmaceuticals for Human Use (ICH) topics "Timing of non-clinical safety studies for the conduct of human clinical trials of pharmaceuticals" and "Pre-clinical safety assessment of biotechnology-derived pharmaceuticals". Conduct of Human Clinical Trials of Pharmaceuticals" and "Preclinical Safety Assessment of Biotechnology-Derived Pharmaceuticals" for studies to be conducted to support the use of therapeutics in humans (Anonymous, 2006).

1.1. Phyto-toxicite

Natural health products (NHPs) may also have indirect adverse effects when used in situations where emergency medical care is required and treatment is delayed. The disclosure of adverse effects (AEs) associated with the use of NHPs is reported to be low (Gillmour et al, 2011; Walji et al, 2010).

The possible risks of negative interactions between natural health products and medicines are often mentioned. In some cases, this possibility is real. However, in many other cases, the opposite is true.

The combination of drugs and natural health products can be beneficial (Guenette et al, 2009). Like their pharmaceutical counterparts in Canada, the majority of NHPs are not tested in the population. In addition, there are few clinical trials and safety data on NHPs. Even when safety studies are available for specific ingredients, the effects of using a combination of multiple ingredients have generally not been studied to a great extent (Murty et al, 2012).

1.1.1. Evaluation procedures

The assessment of toxicity is based on appropriate **qualitative** (non-measurable) or **quantitative** (measurable) studies. There are several types of studies that allow us to assess the effects of a toxicant. They can be classified into four categories: epidemiological studies, which compare several groups of individuals or case studies; *in vivo* experimental studies, which use animals (e.g. rabbits, rats and mice); *in vitro* studies, which use tissue cultures or cells; and theoretical modelling studies (e.g. structure-activity) (Viau and Tardif, 2003). Poor evaluation results can therefore result from a number of factors, ranging from the erroneous use of unsuitable plant species to contamination by toxic substances during storage to overdosing (Coulibaly, 2008).

1.1.2. Hepato toxicity

The liver is a crossroads organ because of the volume of blood that passes through it and because of its privileged location between the digestive tract (portal vein) and the general circulation, making it an essential storage and distribution organ and between the general circulation and the biliary tree, making it an excretory organ (Mekroud, 2004). The liver is the main site of biotransformation of xenobiotics, and any hepatic disease (steatosis, cirrhosis, necrosis) modifies their metabolism and consequently their toxicity (Viala and Botta, 2007). Macroscopic examination (colour, appearance, weight) can indicate the nature of the toxicity and microscopy detects subcellular changes, thus determining the mode of action. Furthermore, the presence of numerous enzymes (Glutamic Pyruvate Transferase (TGP:ALT), Glutamao Oxalo-acetate Transaminase (TGO:ASAT) released from the cytosol and subcellular organelles is evidence of hepatotoxicity (Frank, 1992; Atsamo et al, 2011).

1.1.3. Nephron toxicity

Functional exploration of the kidney consists of statistical and dynamic tests, which can provide valuable information about the integrity of the renal parenchyma (Mekroud, 2004). The renal parenchyma is particularly vulnerable (all areas of the nephron) to a number of toxic substances that can cause damage, ranging from mild biochemical alterations leading to minor dysfunction to cell death leading to renal failure (Cronin and Henrich, 2005).

On histological examination, necrosis of epithelial cells and/or epithelial vacuolation can be found (Richet, 1988)

An elevated blood urea level indicates glomerular damage. Thus an elevated blood creatinine concentration is indicative of renal dysfunction (Frank, 1992).

2. Healing products

Despite the existence of a multitude of healing products with established efficacy, many authors are testing the healing activity of new conventional products, whether they are widely or narrowly used, most often chosen from ethno-pharmaceutical heritages (Bensegueni et al, 2007).

Many plants have been shown to have therapeutic potential as wound healing promoters. *Aloe vera* (Choi et al, 2001*), Centella asiatica* (Suguna et al, 1996*), Pterocarpus angolensis* (Hutchings et al, 1996*), Channa striatus-cetrimide* (Baie and Sheikh, 2000), *Datura alba* (Priya et al, 2002*), Terminalia chebula* (Suguna et al, 2002*), Cinnamomum zeylanicum* (Kamath et al, 2003), *Pterocarpus santalinus* (Biswas et al, 2004), *Butea monosperma* (Sumitra et al, 2005), *Phellinus gilvus* (Bae et al, 2005), *Cassia fistula* (Kumar et al, 2006), *Napoleons imperialis, Ocimum gratissimum and Ageratum conyzoides* (Shah et al, 2006), *Tragic involucrata* (Perumal et al, 2006), *Plagiochasma appendiculatum* (Singh et al, 2006), *Sphaeranthus indicus* (Sadaf et al, 2006), *Tephrosia purpurea* (Lodhi et al, 2006), *Baphia nitida* (Dally et al, 2007), *Embelia ribes* (Kumara Swamy et al, 2007). We have preferred to concentrate on the work carried out in Algeria, especially that carried out at the University of Constantine, the synthesis of which follows.

2.1. *Lawsonia inermis*

Henna has followed the expansion of ISLAM, and has been used in cosmetology for almost 3 millennia for its dyeing properties. Used since ancient times, especially in Egypt and Arabia (Bruneton, 1987), the dyeing properties are due to the energetic fixation of the Lawson on the hair and skin, probably through the reaction with the thiol groups of keratin, a principle used in shampoo and hair lotion. Henna thus gives the skin and hair a mahogany brown colour (Bruneton, 1993). In folk medicine, henna is said to have many diuretic and astringent properties in gastrointestinal ulcers and in the treatment of amoebic diarrhoea (Vanhellement, 1986).

In his work, Ghileb (1987), reports that, in addition to its properties for internal use, henna is used in Morocco, as a poultice, alone or associated with cade tar in eczema and furunculosis, as an external antiseptic and healing agent for wounds and burns.

In Tunisia, henna decoctions are used as antipyretic, antidiarrheal, antidiabetic, hypotensive and in the treatment of oral infections, gingivitis and mouth ulcers. The proven pharmacological virtues of henna include emmenagogic properties, an oxytocic action attributed to lawsone or Lawson and a powerful fungicide (Kerharo and Gadam, 1974; Bruneton, 1993).

In Algeria, work published by Hamdi Pacha et al. (1998a) and (2002), showed a probable effect of *Lawsonia inermis L.* as a wound healer on 3^{ieme} degree burns in rabbits.

Other results showed the positive effect of henna (D17) on healing compared with other plants: cedar of atlas (D20), juniper and *Kniphofia uvularia* (D25), Aleppo pine and *Inula viscosa* (D25), *Centella* (D32) (Hamdi Pacha et al, 1998b). Investigations confirmed the interesting healing effect of the henna plant, in an average time of 17 days compared to a known active principle in Algeria which is madecassol (Benazzouz, 2001).

Using the liquid dilution method, *Pistacia lentiscus* and *Lawsonia inermis* showed antifungal effects on *Trichophyton mentagrophyte* and *Candida albicans* (Mansour Djaaleb et al, 2012).

2.2. *Pistacia lentiscus*

In traditional medicine, pistachio resin is used to combat stomach ulcers. Mastic is often used in medicine as an astringent, expectorant and healing agent (Seigue, 1985).

In Egypt, the resin of the mastic tree, generally called "mastic", was used to embalm the dead, and was later used as a sedative and analgesic, but also as a carminative and diuretic remedy, applied to eczema, boils and other skin conditions, and as a dressing on decayed teeth (Hans Kothe, 2007).

Mastic oils are used for their pharmacological effects as venous decongestant, lymphatic decongestant, antispasmodic. (Baudoux, 2003); they are indicated in the following diseases: varicose veins and heavy legs, congestion and venous stasis, internal and external hemorrhoids, thrombophlebitis, bedsores, cardiac-vascular disorders, rheumatic endocarditis, aerophagia, aerocolia, gastric ulcer, spasmodic colitis, diabetes, sinusitis (decongestant), prostatitis, prostatic congestions and adenomas. (Yahya, 1992; Iserin, 2001; Baudoux, 2003; Grosjean, 2007).

Further results concluded that the fatty oil of the mastic fruit, and in particular its unsaponifiable fraction, has a marked protective and inductive action during the proliferative phase of the excisional wound healing process in rats. This activity is probably associated with the different phytochemical constituents, notably the phytosterols contained in the unsaponifiable fraction (Belfedle, 2009; Boulebda et al, 2009).

Research has been carried out to assess the potential skin, mucous membrane and oral toxicity of mastic as determined by the rabbit safety test and the mouse acute test. The latter test revealed that mastic oil is not toxic in the short term, while the biochemical determination of blood parameters in rabbits treated following rectal administration for six weeks showed that mastic oil can be hepatotoxic in the medium and long term (Boukeloua, 2009).

Further investigations have shown a significant effect of lentisk oil on contraction and reduction of the healing period in rabbits (P<0.05) (Djerrou et al, 2010; Djerrou et al, 2011).

Thus, the comparative study of wound contraction of the two batches (albino rats and wistar strain) showed a significant difference, to the advantage of the batch treated with lentisk oil, results that suggest a healing action of lentisk oil and justify the traditional use of this oil as a wound healer (Abdeldjlil et al, 2012; Abdeldjlil et al, 2014).

It is important to note that the oil is minimally irritating to the eyes and skin after a single exposure, but it can cause irritant contact dermatitis and reversible skin thickening after prolonged use (Djerrou et al, 2013a,b).

2.3. *Argania spinosa*

The Argan tree bears fruit from the age of 5 years but its optimal yield is only reached at the age of 60 years. The study of the composition of the oil in fatty acids, shows that they are more than 80% of oleic, linoleic type. These essential fatty acids confer to the argan oil certain nutritional and dietetic values and justify its use for the cardiovascular diseases and against the diabetes, as well as for the drying and the physiological ageing of the skin (Radi, 2003).

According to Moukal (2004), this "argan oil" is used in the traditional Moroccan pharmacopoeia, in cases of acne and desquamation of the skin, burns and sores, to nourish dry hair, to prevent their fall and to keep their brightness, correcting skin disorders and treating dry and wrinkled skin (anti-wrinkle and anti-ageing effect), aphrodisiac or fortifying, healing of burns and eczema, sprains, wounds or scabies.

The regular application of cosmetological quality argan oil on the skin is recommended for the treatment of chapped, dry or dehydrated skin and acne. In the long term, the application of argan oil leads to a reduction in the speed of appearance of wrinkles and the disappearance of scars caused by measles or chickenpox. The application of argan oil is also recommended for the treatment of superficial burns (Charroufa and Guillaume, 2007).

2.4. *Knifofia uvalaria Moench.*

Results show a positive effect on the healing process by improving the speed of healing and the final appearance of the scar tissue (Hamdi Pacha et al, 1995).

2.5. *Inula viscosa*

There is evidence of a healing effect in *"in vivo"* experiments on 3eme degree burns in rabbits (Chari, 1999; Hamdi Pacha et al, 2002).

2.6. *Juniperus oxycedrus*

The healing effect of cade oil on experimental burns was confirmed by the work of Serakta (1999), carried out on rabbits; the healing of burns treated with the galenic preparation based on cade oil was obtained in 23 days, whereas burns treated with the placebo healed in 27 days.

2.7. *Opuntia ficus indica L.*

The plant can to some extent explain its use in diabetes, a traditional therapy with hypolipidemia, hypoglycemia and anti-obesity effects without any biological toxicity (Halmi et al, 2012, Boukeloua et al, 2012; Halmi et al, 2013). Another study conducted in the pharmaco-toxicology laboratory, on the evaluation of the healing effect of two *Opuntia ficus-indica* products (One, a homogeneous aqueous extract of the paddles and a fine powder of the seeds) following experimental burns, whose results showed a significant reduction of healing times and that *Opuntia ficus-indica.* may possibly stimulate the healing process of second degree burns (Ben Laksira et al, 2013).

2.8. Honey

Honey has antibacterial activity with potent *in vitro* activity against antibiotic resistant bacteria with bactericidal and bacteriostatic power; also healing properties when glucose (from honey) is broken down in the presence of water and oxygen by glucooxidase, gluconic acid and oxygenated water (H_2O_2) are formed.

The oxygenated water formed has a very important role in the healing process. Indeed, it is a very good antiseptic and stimulates the development of neo vascularisation in the scar tissue (Attipou et al, 1998). It has been shown that honey is capable of eliminating certain toxins, especially of fungal origin. In addition, it has an aperitive, anti-anemic and digestive action, antitussive, expectorant and soothing properties, also promotes sleep, is an excellent fuel for the heart muscle, improves blood circulation, fights against chronic constipation, participates in the balance of the neurovegetative system, has antioxidant properties and fights against aging (Rossant, 2011).

Other results confirm the healing effect of honey on the treatment of skin wounds in horses, with complete success in both chronic, heavily budded wounds and fresh wounds (Scohier, 2000).

Thus, research has shown that honey stimulates monocytes to produce inflammatory cytokines, which have an important and favourable role in the inflammatory phase of the wound healing process (Tonks et al, 2003).

Majtan and his team (2010), showed that honey is able to activate the proliferation of keratinocytes (especially during the epithelialization process), by positively regulating the expression of certain cytokines.

Maameri and his team (2012) confirmed in their work that an improvement of the inflammatory phase of the scarring process experienced in laboratory rats is established, if lentisque oil is mixed with honey.

The latest study by Djerrou (2014), proposes the remarkable effects of an ointment, a mixture of bee honey and *Fagopyrum esculentum Moench* seed powder that stimulates the inflammatory phase, the contraction of the wound and the improvement of the healing time.

2.9. Traditional ointment

Investigations confirm the healing activity of two ointments: the first one (pine gum plus onion plus mugwort plus beeswax plus fresh butter) and the second one (beeswax plus mastic oil) which is recognised in the folk medicine of the Constantine region, Algeria (Bensegueni, 2007).

2.10. Fresh yeast plus bramble leaves

Among the treated batches, the fourth batch of laboratory rats (mixture of butter and bramble leaf powder) showed the best evolution of their scars (Kaddour and Haouam, 2010).

3. Hair stimulants

Natural products have been allowed to spread in the hair care industry and almost a thousand kinds of plant extracts have been examined with regard to hair growth promoting activity, some of them, thus, have shown a huge potential. Polyherbal compounds are generally used as hair tonic, hair growth promoter, conditioner, hair washing agent, as well as for the treatment of alopecia and lice infection and are created as a realistic and safe option without side effects for men and women facing their hair loss problem (Roy et al, 2008; Patil et al, 2010).

3.1. Procyanidin B-2

It is a polyphenolic compound (extracted from apples and grapes) with activity on hair, causing a modulation of the expression and translocation of Proteine Kinase C isoenzymes which act negatively on hair epithelial cells. The results, combined with those of other investigations, suggest a possible link between the hair growth activity possessed by procyanidin B-2 and its down-regulation or inhibition of translocation of PKC isoenzymes in hair epithelial cells in addition to its PKC inhibitory activity. It is highly likely that PKC plays a key role in hair and hair cycle regulation (Kamimura and Takahashi, 2002).

3.2. *Hibiscus rasa sinensis Linn*

Adhirajan and his team (2003) prove that *Hibiscus rasa sinensis L.* leaf extract stimulates better hair follicle activity in rats compared to flowers.

3.3. *Asiasari radix*

In 2005, Rho's team confirmed that *Asiasari radix* extract is a good candidate for promoting hair growth.

3.4. Mixing of oils

The mixture of oils (Amla, Brahim, Methi and Meeth Neem) significantly increased hair growth activity in rabbits compared to the standard and is becoming a potential alternative to Minoxidil (Purwal et al, 2008; Pooja et al, 2009).

3.5. Raspberry Acetone

Topical application of 0.01% raspberry acetone increases IGFI (Insulin like Growth Factor- 1), produced by the hair follicles of the sensory neuron, and promises hair growth in men with alopecia (Harda et al, 2008).

3.6. *Eclipta alba*

The results of the treatment with 2 and 5% petroleum ether extracts of *Eclipta alba* were better than the positive treatment with 2% Minoxidil control regarding hair growth in albino rats (Roy et al, 2008).

3.7. *Prunus dulcis*

Prunus dulcis seeds have been traditionally known for hair growth activity, which is proven by the work of Suraj and his team in 2009:Petroleum ether, methanol, chloroform and water extracted from *Prunus dulcis* seeds incorporated in the oleaginous ointment base were applied topically to the shaved skin of albino rats tested for hair growth activity

3.8. *Russelia equisetiformis*

Experimental data obtained in the animal study by Awe and Makinde in (2009) indicate that the crude methanol extract *Russelia equisetiformis* has hair growth promoting potential.

3.9. *Zizyphus jujuba*

The efficacy of 1% *Zizyphus jujuba* seed oil and its potential role on hair growth *in vivo was* demonstrated after 21 days of application to mice by Yoon and his team in 2010.

3.10. *Tamarindus indica* and *Curcuma longa*

The study by Vyas et al (2010) to evaluate the effect of *Tamarindus indica* and *Curcuma longa* on alopecia-induced stress is very promising.

3.11. *Abrus precatorius*

The work of Upadhyay and his team in 2012(a) concluded that the ethanolic extract of *Abrus precatorius L.* seeds has anti androgenic activity and can cause alopecia due to inhibition of the enzyme 5a- reductase.

3.12. Glycyrrhiza. Glabra

Oil ether root extract from Glycyrrhiza. Glabra is more effective than Minoxidil in promoting hair growth in female Wistar rats. The herbal extract would be preferred, not only because of its natural origin, but also because Minoxidil has several side effects (Upadhyay et al, 2012 b).

3.13. *Allium sativum*

Whole, chopped or crushed garlic has been used for centuries in medicine and cooking for its tonic properties (Iserin, 2001).

Garlic has antiseptic, bactericidal, expectorant, stimulant, vermifuge and hypotensive properties. The medicinal effect is due to the bulb. It is also used as an anticancer and antidiabetic. Garlic is effective against venom, hemorrhoids, loss of voice and kidney ailments. It has been rightly considered as a preservative against infectious diseases: cholera, typhus, typhoid, diphtheria (Beloued, 2009).

Garlic is also beneficial for the hair, it stops hair loss and promotes hair growth, it is composed of "sulphur". Sulphur is a component of "keratin" which makes the hair stronger; it also improves the condition of the scalp. Garlic contains vitamin B6, also vitamin C which makes the root stronger and therefore helps to stop hair loss, vitamin B1 which promotes blood circulation and allows regrowth (Anonymous, 2012).

CHAPTER IV:
MONOGRAPHY OF
LINUM USSITATISSIMUM

1. General

Flax or linseed, is one of the oldest plants cultivated (Figure 7) for its oil and fibre. The botanical name, *Linum usitatissimum* was given by Linnaeus in 1857 in his book "Species Plantarum" (Cited by Jhalla and Hall, 2010).

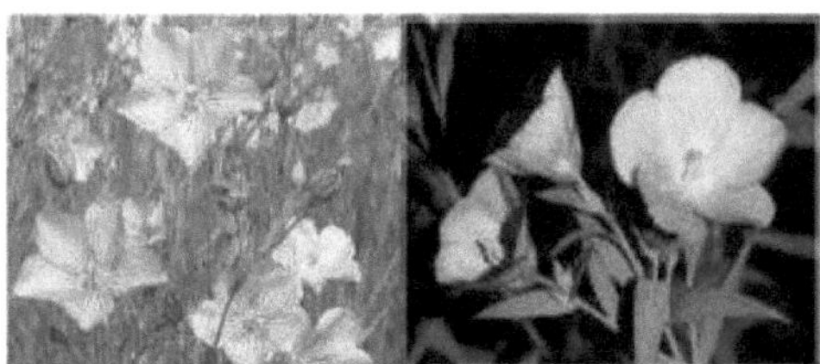

Figure 7: Blue flower of *Linum usitatissimum* (Heli et al, 2007)

The use of flax by humans has been documented for over 30,000 years. The plant is native to Western Asia and the Mediterranean (Millam et al, 2005), cultivated as a source of fibre since at least 5000 BC, it became mainly cultivated for its oil (Oomah, 2001; Berugland, 2002).

Its Latin name '*Linum usitatissimum*' (flax of all uses) is well deserved (Weill and Mairesse, 2010).

It is a rare plant in its spontaneous state and is cultivated as a textile or oilseed crop depending on the variety considered (Diederichsen *et* al, 2003; Vaisey-Genser et al, 2003). There are about 180 varieties of cultivated flax (*Linum usitatissimum L*) in the EU, including about 60 in France, registered in the official French and European catalogues. There are more than 200 cultivated varieties in the list of the Organisation for Economic Co-operation and Development (OECD), intended for international trade. Worldwide, there are about 10,000 pure lines or ecotypes held in collections (Anonymous, 2010).

Annual flax production is 3.06 million tonnes. Canada is the largest producer of flax, accounting for about 38% of world production, followed by China, the USA, India and the EU (Jhalla and Hall, 2010, Rubilar et al, 2010, Ganorkar and Jain, 2013).

2. Botanical description

It is a self-pollinating dicotyledonous plant that belongs to the Linaceae family and the genus Linum (Bloedon and Szapary, 2004). Flax is an annual, biennial or perennial plant, extremely slender, rather shallowly rooted (taproot) as flax is uprooted, not mown (Roberto, 1982; Bernard, 2001). This plant grows to a maximum height of 60 cm, with elongated forms and very fibrous stems, lanceolate leaves with three veins, up to 4 cm long and 4 mm wide and its bright blue flowers are up to 3 cm in diameter (Pradhan et al, 2010). The spherical fruit capsules contain two seeds in each of the five compartments. The seed is flat and oval with a pointed tip (Figure 8). It has a smooth and shiny surface. Its colour varies from dark brown to yellow (Freeman, 1995). The texture of the flaxseed is crunchy and soft with a pleasant nutty taste (Carter, 1996).

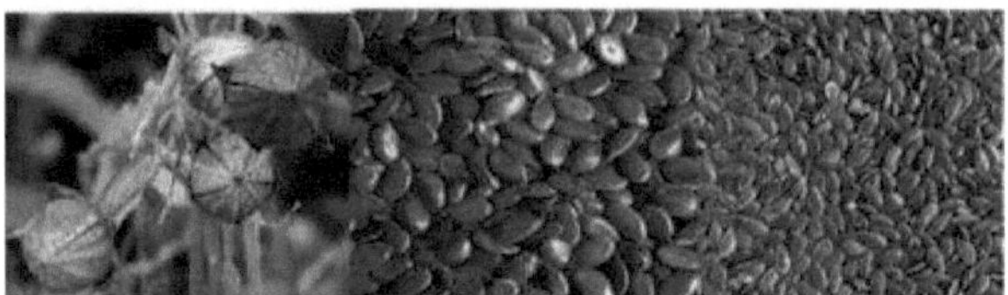

Figure 8: Flaxseed and fruit (Heli et al, 2007; Halligudi, 2012).

In addition to the cultivated species, there are also wild flax species (Figure 9). Yellow flax, *Linum flavum*, is a biennial yellow-flowered species that occurs naturally in Central and Eastern Europe and Northern Italy. It has a single stem and a five-petal yellow flower. Other wild flaxes include *Linum angustifolium*, the probable ancestor of cultivated flax; *Linum album*, a white-flowered flax endemic to Iran; *Linum grandiflorum*, a species of southern flax of African origin with large red flowers; and *Linum perenne, which occurs* in Europe and temperate Asia and is a rounded clump. Ornamental varieties exist for *Linum grandiflorum* and *Linum perenne*. There are also other species of yellow-flowered flax including *Linum nodiflorum* (Renouard, 2011).

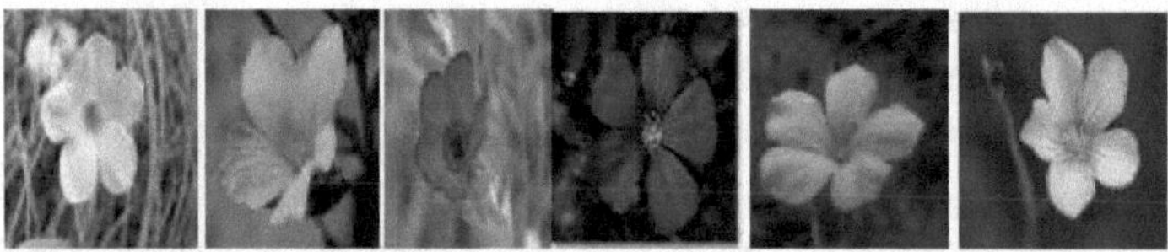

Linum album Linum Flavum Linum grandiflorum Linum perenne Linum nodiflorum Linum angustifolium
Figure 9: Wild flax *(*Renouard, 2011).

3. Composition

Flaxseed oil is unique because it is composed of 73% polyunsaturated fatty acids (PUFAs), 18% monounsaturated fatty acids (MUFAs) and 9% saturated fatty acids (SFAs), making it a low-saturated fat food (Table II). It is also known to be the richest source of omega-3 (n-3) fatty acids, ALA, which comprises 55% of total fatty acids (Appendix 1). The percentage of ALA in flaxseed oil is 5.5 times higher than that of walnuts and canola oil (Heli et al, 2007).

Table II: Fatty acids in flaxseed oil (Morris, 2003 cited by Ganorkar and Jain, 2013)

Parameters	Percentage (%)
Saturated Fatty Acid	9
AG Mono insature	18
Linoleic acid (omega-6)	16

The seed contains about 40% fat, 30% dietary fibre and 20% protein (Table III). It is rich in lipids, mainly unsaturated oils: alphalinolenic acid (ALA) or omega-3 (Appendix 2). The name linoleic comes from the German lein ol (linseed oil).

The chemical composition varies considerably between varieties and also depends on the environmental conditions in which the plant is grown. The cotyledons contain 75% lipids and 76% of the protein is found in the seeds. The endosperm contains only 23% of the lipid and 16% of the protein (Daun et al, 2003; Oomah, 2003).

Table III: Chemical composition (%) of flaxseed (Rubilar et al, 2010)

Humidity	Protein	Lipid	Fibre	Ash	References
7,4	23,4	45,2	-	3,5	Mueller et al (2010)
4-8	20-25	30-40	20-25	3-4	Coskuner and Karababa (2007)

4. Bioactive molecule

The biological activity of flax lignans is often attributed to their conversion to the mammalian lignans enterolactone and enterodiol (Muir, 2006). Intermediate compounds generated during the digestion and metabolism of flax lignans, such as secoisolariciresinol diglycoside (SDG), its aglycone and secoisolariciresinol (Seco) may also be the main bioactive molecule.

The plant (seed and oil) contains polyunsaturated fatty acids (PUFA), including alpha-linolenic acid (ALA) and linoleic acid. It is poorly converted by the human body to eicosapentaenoic acid (EPA) and decosahexaenoic acid (DHA) (lack of necessary enzymes). Flaxseed also contains monounsaturated fatty acids (MUFA), such as oleic acid. Both ALA and linoleic acid are essential fatty acids (EFAs), which means that they cannot be synthesised by the human body and must be obtained from the diet (Dyerberg, 1986; Slguel, 1994; Stoll et al, 1999), ALA is a precursor of EPA (Mantzioris et al, 1995) and ingestion of flaxseed has been shown to increase cellular EPA levels in a linear fashion (Mantzioris et al, 1994).

However, the linoleic component of flax (e.g. omega-6 fatty acids) has an antagonistic effect on the conversion of ALA to EPA. Flax is a concentrated food source of the lignan SDG. Flaxseed also contains small amounts of the lignans matairesinol (Hutchins et al, 2001), SDG and matairesinol can be converted to mammalian lignans such as enterodiol and enterolactone by colonic bacteria (Rickard et al, 1996).

Apart from its use as an oilseed crop, the composition of flaxseed shows promise for use in various food products (Figure 10). Flaxseed is one of the richest plant sources of a -linolenic acid (omega-3 fatty acids) and soluble mucilage (Ganorkar and Jain, 2013).

5. Therapeutic use

Omega-3 polyunsaturated fatty acids have two main uses:

- The first is their quantitative importance and their role in the development and maintenance of various organs, especially the brain.

- The second is the prevention of various pathologies and cardiovascular diseases (Bourre, 2004; Bloedon and Szapary, 2004).

Flaxseed oil and flaxseed are being rediscovered as real health foods. They deserve to be classified as a life-saving food. Flax is not a new food. It is, in fact, one of the oldest and perhaps one of the original "valuable foods because of its healing properties", a thousand-year-old plant with medicinal properties (Halligudi, 2012).

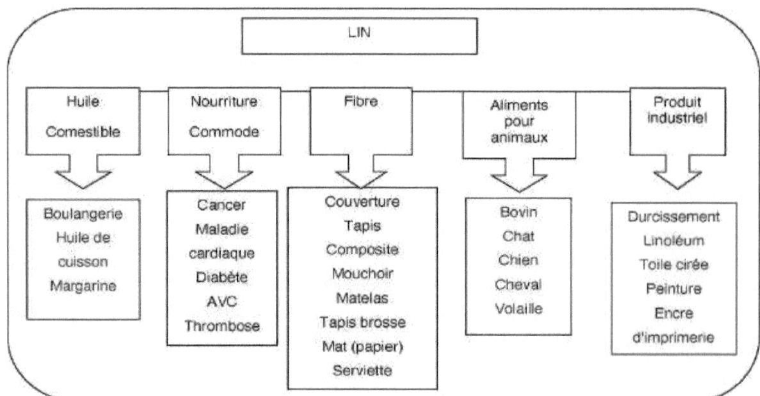

Figure 10: Flax use diagram (Jhalla and Hall, 2010).

5.1. Seeds

Mucilages are polysaccharides which have a very important swelling capacity in a humid environment; it is to them that flaxseed owes its laxative and emollient capacities cited in numerous treatises.

Particularly in cases of chronic constipation in crushed form, its seeds absorb intestinal fluids (Blumenthal et al, 2000). The mucilages promote colonic drainage and help to soften the stool and facilitate its evacuation. Also due to the mucilages, they provide a calming and anti-inflammatory effect reducing colon irritation in conditions such as colitis, intestinal inflammation and hemorrhoids (Iserin, 2001; Halligudi, 2012).

It is perhaps relevant to highlight its properties, at a time when it is sometimes fashionable to use flaxseed to benefit from nutritional claims of the omega-3 type. Although the digestibility of these raw seeds is extremely low, flaxseed also contains lignans which belong to the phytoestrogen family; these lignans have anti-oxidant and anti-cancer properties (Prasad, 1997; Prasad, 2000; Chen et al, 2002; Thompson, 2003; Zanwar et al, 2010). Ingestion of the seed as prevention of breast, uterine and prostate cancer and possibly protection against recurrence (Boon et al, 2007; Heli et al, 2007; Halligudi, 2012).

The seed is also considered to be effective in respiratory and urinary disorders and should be opened before swallowing (Iserin, 2001). It calms lung pain and to a lesser extent irritation of the urinary tract. It is effective against chronic and acute coughs, bronchitis, emphysema and chronic cystitis, as well as being a useful preventive against angina, colds and arteriosclerosis. Thus to reduce postprandial blood glucose and cholesterol levels (Kim and Choi, 2005; Vijaimohan et al, 2006; Halligudi, 2012).

Externally, a poultice of crushed flaxseed or flaxseed meal applied to boils and carbuncles calms ulcers and drains pus (Singh and Majumdar, 1997; Iserin, 2001). In the past, women boiled flax seeds in water and used flax in the form of a gel to soften their hair (Halligudi, 2012). Finally, it is necessary not to use immature flaxseed as it can be toxic (Iserin, 2001). Flaxseed also contains anti-nutritional factors intended to defend them from birds; these factors belong to the cyanogen family (Mazza and Oomah, 1995; Hermier et al, 2004).

5.2. Oil

Linseed oil or linseed oil is a golden yellow oil, extracted from the ripe seeds of the cultivated flax plant, cold and/or hot pressed; sometimes it is extracted by a solvent, for industrial or artistic use, mainly as a siccative, or self-drying oil as a mastic for caulking and sealing. Linseed oil is used for painting and varnishing, for saturating slate material, for developing black soap and for protecting coins as well as rusty steel. It is impregnated and protects the wood inside and outside: protection against moisture, fungi and insects and against dust by its antistatic character. Linseed oil has a thick to liquid texture and is light in colour (Bloedon and Szapary, 2004).

It is recommended for people suffering from multiple sclerosis or diabetes. It also has an effect on the hormonal and immune systems. Daily use of linseed oil protects the gastric and urinary membrane. Linseed oil is also suitable for face, body (massage and body care). Externally, the oil obtained from the seeds is known for its softening and emollient properties. It protects and softens irritated skin (Halligudi, 2012).

Flaxseed oil is also used in diets for pets, including dogs, cats and horses. The essential fatty acids (ALA and LA) present in flaxseed contribute to a glossy coat, help prevent dry skin and dandruff and also help reduce digestive and skin problems in animals (Jhalla and Hall, 2010). It is also used in the treatment of hides, to nourish horses' hooves (Blumenthal et al, 2000; Bloedon and Szapary, 2004). Flaxseed oil is not an interesting source of omega-3 intake, even though the oils are considered to be anti-oxidant and stored in opaque packages away from light; they would be rapidly beta-oxidised once ingested (Nelson and Chamberlain, 1995). It should be noted that the same amount of linseed oil from either extruded seeds (moderate cooking and mechanical action replicating traditional preparation methods) or from the mixture of meal and oil provides opposite effects (hypercholesterolemic for the meal and oil; hypocholesterolemic for the extruded seed).

Flaxseed oil has antimicrobial activity against *Staphylococcus aureus; Streptococcus agalactiae, Enterococcus faecalis, Micrococcus luteus, Bacillus subtilis and Candida albicans* (Kaithwas et al, 2011).

6. Effect on zootechnical performance

Cooked linseed introduced into animal nutrition improves animal health and fertility parameters. Clinical studies show that its benefits are not limited to improving the health status of the animals, but give animal products consumed by humans a better nutritional quality: meat, butter, milk, cheese and eggs (Renouard, 2011).

This effect is more important in monogastrics than in polygastrics. For example, the hydrogenating intestinal bacteria of the latter transform a significant fraction of the polyunsaturated fatty acids present in their diet into saturated fatty acids. In practice, the addition of omega-3 fatty acids in the form of flaxseed extracts and their oils to animal feed yields significant results for poultry and rabbits, but very modest results for cattle and sheep (Bourre, 2004). These results are explained by the fact that there are species-related differences in meat composition, as ruminant meat is always richer in saturated fatty acids than monogastric meat. Conversely, chicken and rabbit meat are always richer in n-6 fatty acids than ruminant meat (Chesneau et al, 2004).

6.1. Cattle

Beef is nutritionally rich in saturated fatty acids (fatty products). To produce meat enriched in fatty acids, nutritionists in France recommend n-3 polyunsaturated fatty acids (n-3 PUFA or Omega 3) (Martin, 2001). In cattle, the majority of dietary fatty acids are hydrogenated in the rumen and are therefore poorly incorporated into the products. However, in dairy cows, lipid supplementation of the diet can significantly modulate the lipid composition of milk (Brunschwig et al, 1997; Chilliard et al, 2000).

The results of the study carried out in steers at the end of fattening confirm that supplementation of rations with n-3 polyunsaturated fatty acids (flax) strongly stimulates muscle synthesis and development in beef cattle at the end of fattening

(Bauchart et al, 2002). Vegetable oils added to rations in different forms would enrich beef with polyunsaturated fatty acids and may have an impact on product quality (Clinquart et al, 1995; Bauchart et al, 2001; Durand et al, 2001).

The results of the study by Martin and his team (2007) showed that early fattening bulls fed the extruded linseed supplemented ration ingest less dry matter but the net energy content is higher. They produce less methane. There is no influence of the ration on rumen pH (Eugene et al, 2009).

6.2. Sheep and lamb

Grass grazing and flaxseed supplementation in lambs significantly increase the proportions of C18:3n-3 and conjugated linoleic acids (CLA) and decrease the ratio of n-6/n-3 polyunsaturated fatty acids. Supplementation of the ewe's diet with linseed during the lactation period significantly influences the fatty acid composition of the lambs' meat when the duration of the supplementation is sufficiently long (at least 2/3 of the lamb's life span) and when the time of slaughter of the lambs is not too far from weaning (less than 6 weeks).

In male lambs, the proportion of C18:3n-3 and polyunsaturated fatty acids in meat tends to be higher. On the farm, the meat of male lambs has a significantly higher proportion of CLA than that of females (Rondia et al, 2003).

6.3. Poultry

Farming factors have a strong influence on the quality of the meat, especially the nutritional value (Mourot, 2008). These factors are related to genetics, physiology and farming practices (feeding, free range, management). They influence the nutritional quality of the meat: turkey and chicken legs and fillets.

The seed is used in animal feeds, especially for laying hens where it is desired to increase the w-3 content of the eggs (Table IV). The lipid content of the different chicken and turkey tissues was not significantly influenced by the nature of the diets. However, there is a difference associated with the nature of the tissues; fillets are less rich in lipids than thighs for all species. In the thighs of chickens fed extruded linseed, the proportion of monounsaturated fatty acids decreased significantly ($p < 0.05$); the proportion of polyunsaturated fatty acids was influenced by the nature of the diet, with the latter increasing. The fraction of n-3 fatty acids is higher when animals consume flax (Guillevic et al, 2010).

Table IV: Comparison of fat profile of w-3 enriched and regular eggs
(Canadian Egg Marketing Agency, 2007) (in Jhalla and Hall 2010).

	Enriched sufs w-3	Ordinary sufs
Total fatty acids	4,9 g	5,0 g
w-6	0,7	0,7 g
w-3	0,4 g	0,04 g
Monosature	1,6 g	2,0 g
Saturation	1,2 g	1,5 g
Cholesterol	185 mg	190 mg

6.4. Rabbit

In the medical world, rabbit meat has a positive image because it is reputed to be low or fat-free (Ouhayoun, 1989). As with all monogastric animals, the nutritional quality of the fatty acids in rabbit meat is related to the nature of the lipids that the animal ingests (Colin et al, 2005; Mourot, 2010). Even if rabbit meat does not represent an important part of the consumption of meat products, an increase in the content of n-3 fatty acids in rabbit meat can contribute to the supply of more of these fatty acids in the human diet (Dalle Zotte, 2000, Weill et al, 2004, Colin et al, 2005, Kouba et al, 2008, Benatmane et al, 2010).

The study by Dumas and his team (2003) shows that the addition of extruded linseed to rabbit feed is likely to increase the Omega-3 fatty acid content of shoulder, thigh, spleen and liver muscles without altering the hedonic characteristics.

PROBLEMATICS

Presentation

Burns are one of the most frequent reasons for consultation in emergency departments. This serious danger can pose complex therapeutic problems. In folk medicine, however, there are plants that are used with good reputation in the healing process and that should be evaluated in this field of research. One of the objectives of this work is to confront the action of *Linum ussitatissimum* (j^l) with the phenomenon of epithelial regeneration.

Another problem as painful as the first one is represented by alopecia or hair loss, which is not only an aesthetic problem, but also a psychosociological one. A therapeutic strategy is being explored for the promotion of hair growth with flax. Indeed, it is also known in traditional medicine as a medication for hair loss. It is in this second context that our work has been selected and its interest

However, exploring herbal medicines is based on a more scientific indication. This can be achieved by demonstrating real efficacy in in *vivo* experiments on laboratory animals (Albino rabbits) and finally by demonstrating their safety. In the present study, the safety of the seed was demonstrated during the evaluation of hair growth.

As for new raw materials for animal feed, flax (source of Omega 3 fatty acids) has consistently proven its value.

The impact of flaxseed on the zootechnical performance of rabbits is the last question addressed in the experimental study.

Objectives:
1. General
In the present study, the main objective is to find out the pharmacological value of flax (*Linum usitatissimum*).
2. Specific :
*To evaluate the action of *Linum usitatissimum* oil on epithelial regeneration (healing of experimental burns).
*To assess the effect and effectiveness of the plant (seed and its extracted oil) on the hair system (hair growth**)**.
*Control the safety of repeated and prolonged ingestion of the seed.
*To know the impact of seed supplementation on some zootechnical performances of adult rabbits.

EXPERIMENTAL PROTOCOL

The experimental part is formed by two examinations, the first is preclinical (*in vivo*), carried out in the animal house of the laboratory of pharmacotoxicology, of the Institute of Veterinary Sciences, University Mentourie Constantine 1, the second is para-clinical (*in vitro*) and carried out in collaboration with a laboratory of biochemistry and histology. In order to meet the set objectives, the adult male Neo-Zealand rabbit is selected to carry out all the tests (during 9 months). The chosen experimental model has a sufficiently large back surface for four skin burns and is also a good model for the study of hair growth.

Handling is done at the same time to avoid stressing the rabbits. The entire procedure is adopted in accordance with the International Ethical Guidelines for the Care and Use of Laboratory Animals in Research and Education (FELASA, 2007).

The experimental protocol involves the study of the pharmacological activity of linseed oil and linseed. It is carried out according to the following scheme (Figure 11):

• **A**: consists of provoking experimental burns in rabbits and treating them daily, for 04 weeks, with an application of linseed oil. The action of the oil on epithelial regeneration is compared with other products tested. It is assessed by the evolution of the diameter of the wound surfaces and their appearance on histological examination.

• **B**: dedicated to estimate the effect of oil on hair growth in rabbits. The length, diameter and weight of the hair are the parameters measured.

• **C**: consists of daily supplementation of the rabbits' feed ration with ground flaxseed for 13 consecutive weeks. Three effects are then estimated:

• **C1**: hair growth. The same parameters described above are measured every month.

• **C2**: safety of the seed by repeated ingestion. Monitoring (clinical, biochemical and histological) is instituted.

• **C3**: zootechnical performance of the adult rabbit. Average daily gain and slaughter yield are recorded

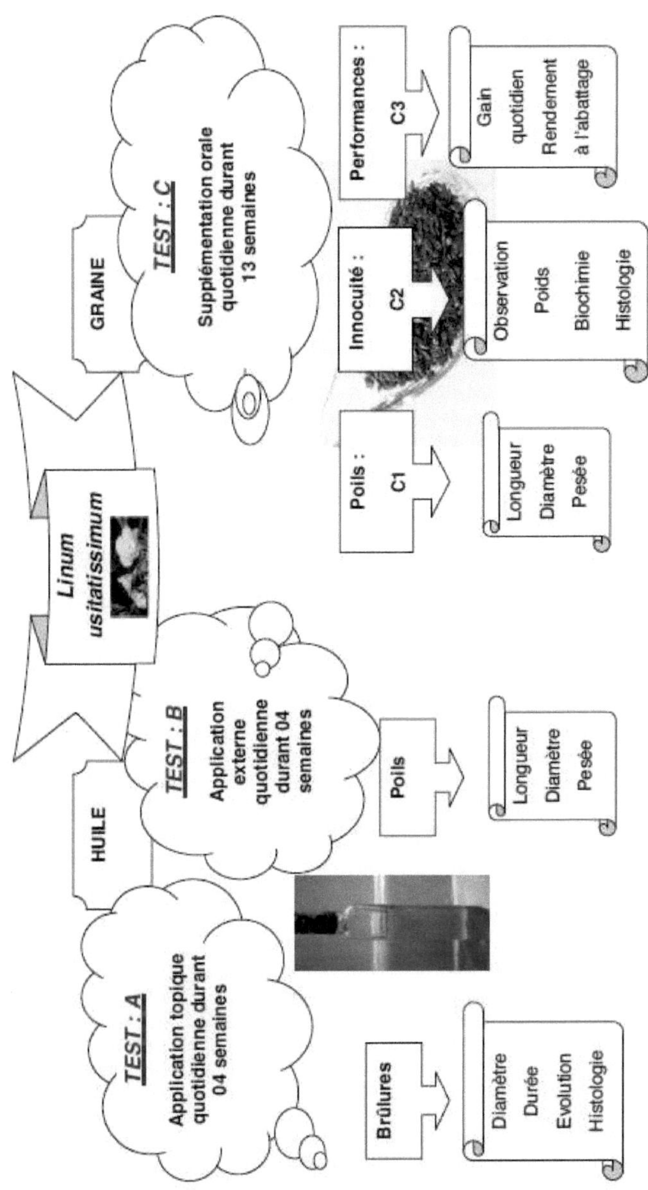

Figure 11: Experimental protocol

CHAPTER V :
EVALUATION OF
EPITHELIAL REGENERATION

The study of wound healing, which is a dynamic and interactive biological process, can be done either by studying lesions of various and accidental origins or by monitoring experimental lesions induced in healthy laboratory animals. Due to the high variability of lesions in the former case, comparison of results is difficult from one lesion to another, hence the need to induce experimental lesions in a standardised manner. Standardisation of the size of the induced lesions allows comparison of the healing process and the factors that may influence it (Ferraq, 2007).

In order to evaluate the effect of linseed oil *(Linum usitatissimum)* on epithelial regeneration. The procedure for this part is to apply linseed oil and other substances (tested separately for comparison) daily to heal the wounds. The healing effect is studied by daily monitoring of the evolution of the diameters of the contraction surfaces of the burns, by observation of clinical variation and completed by histological examination of the wound.

1. MATERIALS AND METHODS

1.1. Animals

Homogenous batches of adult (albino) rabbits from a single animal house in Ain M'Lila (north of Algiers) were used for the study. The animals were of male sex and of more or less identical weight at the start of the experimental protocol (3000g±0.5). They were marked twice a week to preserve their identity in each batch. Their numbers varied from 06 to 12 for each test. The animals are placed in individual cages equipped with a feeder, a bottle of water and a label holder where the name of the batch, the treatment undergone and the dates of handling are mentioned. The cages are stored in a battery, in a standardised environment, with an ambient temperature of 22-32°C and a natural light-dark cycle. The bedding used is sawdust, changed twice a week.

Feed and water are provided *ad libitum*. The feed distributed to the rabbits is standard "CEREGRAIN" composed of: alfalfa, barley, maize, soya, CCV (vitamin complex).

1.2 Burning technique

The approach is carried out (Figure 12) in accordance with the technique described by Hamdi Pacha et al (2002):

1. The backs of the rabbits are clipped with an electric clipper and a razor blade 24 hours before the start of the test (figure 12A).

2. On day zero, all rabbits are anaesthetised with ketamine hydrochloride by intramuscular injection (1ml/10kg).

3. The four areas to be burned are locally anaesthetised with xylocaine infiltration at a dose of 1ml per burn (Figure 12B).

4. Four burns are made on each side of the dorsolumbar spine of each rabbit.

5. A 200g, 2cm diameter club is held for 3 minutes in boiling water (100°C). It is immediately dried and placed on the rabbit's skin for 15 seconds without exerting force (Figure 12C).

6. After the metal piece has cooled down, the other burns are carried out in the same way. Each animal has its own control. Each of the wounds receives a specific treatment (tests or control). Wound diameters are taken every other day (figure 12 E).

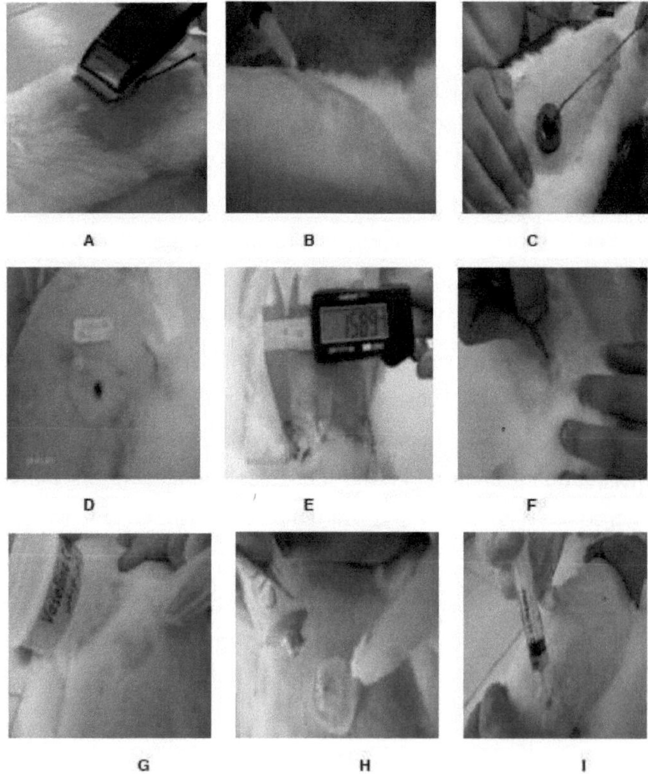

Figure 12: Stages of the experimental burns.

A: Shaved rabbit back, **B**: Anaesthetised area, **C**: Warm sledgehammer applied, **D**: Burnt area identified, **E**: Diameter measurement, **F**: Margin of a wound traced on transparent paper, **G**: Application of Vaseline, H: Treated with Cicatryl-Bio, I: Treatment with linseed oil
G: Application of Vaseline, **H**: Treated with Cicatryl-Bio, **I**: Treatment with linseed oil.

1.3. Wound treatment

Immediately after the burns are made, the test products are applied topically, as indicated below:

Burn 1: no product, natural healing, (NAT).

Burn 2: treated with Vaseline 1g/314cm^2, (placebo: VAS, Figure 12G)

Burn 3: application of 1g/314cm2 of Cicatryl-Bio, (CIC, figure 12H)

Burn 4: treated with linseed oil at a dose of 1ml/314cm2, (HL, figure 12I).

The wound treatment is rotational, each product is applied to the dorsal and lumbar region in six rabbits. All products are administered once a day until complete epithelialisation is observed.

1.4. Assessment of wound healing

The evaluation of the healing process has several approaches such as: clinical, physical, biochemical, and histological. The study adopted morphological parameters, including wound surface, epithelialization period and histological approach.

1.4.1. Observation of wounds

The macroscopic appearance (appearance, colour, odour) and external evolution of the wound are examined and noted daily before the application of the healing products during the entire treatment period.

1.4.2. Planimetric study

Wound margins are marked on transparent paper and the horizontal and vertical diameters of each wound are measured every other day with an electronic caliper (accuracy 0.001mm).

The average wound area is calculated according to the formula: R2 xn, where R is the radius (the average of the two diameters of each area).

The percentage of wound contraction is calculated every four days (D_4, D_8, D_{12}, D_{16}, D_{20}, D_{24}, D_{28}), using the formula of Srivastava and Durgaprasad (2008): Percentage wound contraction= [(initial wound area - specific day's wound area) / initial wound area] x 100.

The initial area is 314cm^2, with a diameter of 2cm.

Photographs of the wounds are taken every other day, to create a real picture of the chronology of the burns and the progress of the healing process.

1.5. Observation and weight gain

Clinical changes in the rabbits were noted regularly. Observation included general condition, mortality and any other changes (appetite, behaviour, signs of pain and faecal condition).

At the end of each week and at the same time, the rabbits are weighed using an ordinary scale (NEW CROWN, D: 0.01, Max: 30Kg), before the feed is distributed. The individual body weight of the animals is recorded on an individual sheet (Appendix 6).

1.6. Statistical analysis

Data on average wound diameters and areas as well as average animal weights are calculated in Excel.

The results are statistically analysed using Student's *t-test.*

For all other parts of the study, the results are statistically analysed using the Matlab v7.7.0.2162 (Release 2008b) program. Various tests are applied including Student's *t-test.* The comparison of two means in the case of small samples (<30) is carried out, except in cases where the required conditions are not met (normal population, equality of variances), the non-parametric Wilcoxon test is then used.

1.7. Histological examination

1.7.1. Collection and fixing of parts

On the 35eme day of healing, the rabbits are sacrificed and the 24 samples of regenerated areas are taken in the form of a balloon. The harvested parts are washed and put in labelled pillboxes. They are covered with 10% formalin and stored until use.

1.7.2. Technical

The histological examination is carried out according to the standard technique at the laboratory of pathological anatomy and cytology of Professor Haouam S of Constantine (figure 13). The steps are as follows:

- **Preparation of cuts**

At the macroscopic level, the piece recovered from the formalin is carefully inspected (number, shape, measurements, features) and noted on an identification sheet.

The specimen is washed thoroughly under running water. The cassette with the same sample identification number is opened. Using a board and scalpel, cuts are made in two planes (longitudinal and perpendicular) (Figure 13A). The sections made are placed in the corresponding cassette and immediately closed.

- **Treatment programme**

Ten or so cassettes, placed in the basket, will undergo a succession of timed passes through tanks of solvents (alcohol, xylene) and paraffin (dehydration, thinning, impregnation) (Figure 13B). Consistency in procedure is important to obtain comparable and related test results. The times specified for the steps in the protocol can be modified to suit the specific reagents which may vary slightly in strength and composition (Appendix 7).

- **Inclusion / embedding**

Embedding of the impregnated tissue in a paraffin block is performed using an Embedding Center Tissue Tek device (Figure 13C).

- **Freezing cassettes**

This is the cooling of the paraffin blocks.

- **Roughing and spreading**

The blocks are passed through a rotary microtome (Leica RM2125RTS.Applications-R) (with disposable razors) to obtain films of each sample (Figure 13D), for spreading on a slide referenced by the same identification number (Figure 13: E-F). The slides are dried on a hot plate (Figure 13G).

- **Colouring**

Slides stored in the slide holder will undergo a succession of timed passes through trays of solvents and stains (hematoxylin, eosin) according to the standard Hemalun Eosin stain (Figure 13: H-I) followed by a series of ringing and draining (Appendix 8)

- **Assembly and labelling**

Each slide is covered with a fixed coverslip using mounting fluid (Eukit) (Figure 13J-K). The slides are labelled and referenced by the same number (Figure 13).

1.7.3 Interpretation

Histological sections of the various wounds are read and interpreted. The parameters retained are the presence of inflammatory cells, epithelialization of the epidermis, the extent of fibrosis, the presence of granulation tissue and the detection of abnormalities.

The microphotographs were taken with an optical microscope (Leica DME, 85-265.VAC No. 421063938EZ0006) equipped with a digital camera (Nikon COOLPIX S3000).

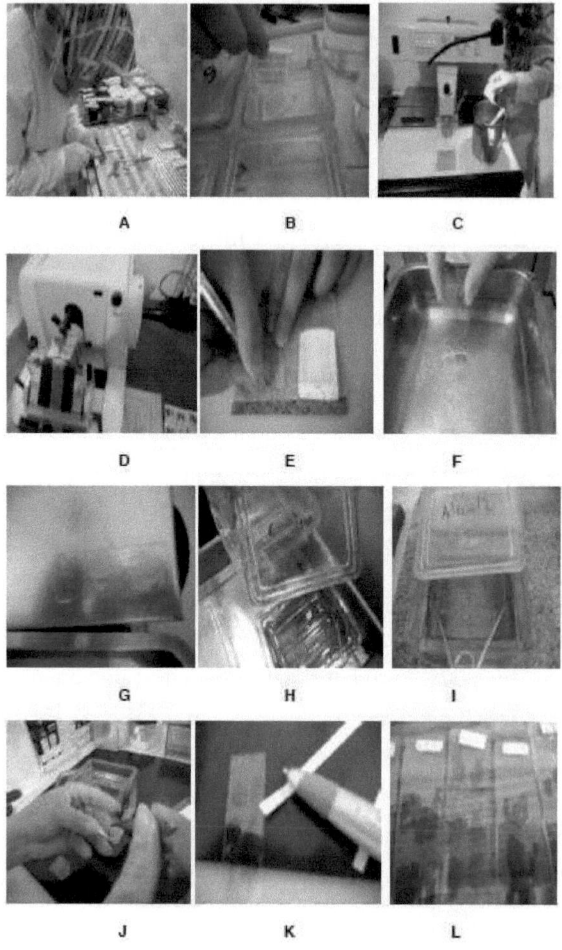

Figure 13: Steps in the pathology study

A: Cassette preparation, **B:** Solvent treatment, **C**: Paraffin embedding

D : Degaussing, **E** : Reference of the slide, **F** : Spreading, **G** : Drying, **H :** Dyeing, **I :** Solvent treatment, **J** : Mounting of the slide, **K** : Labelling, **L** : Filing.

2. RESULTS

2.1. Planimetric study

2.1.1. Wound surface

The different areas obtained are presented in table V, they represent *the mean ± standard deviation, calculated for 06 rabbits treated with the same products for more than 28 days.

Table V: Wound area at different intervals $(cm)^2$

	NAT	VAS	CIC	HL	P
J4	395,26±81,78	345,40±30,56	326,56±25,98	332,87±20,63	NS
J8	418,12±127,41	**254,58±50,66***	255,66±60,54	347,63±77,91	Its
J12	382,35±118,18	**211,64±20,68***	237,35±50,88	320,36±34,15	Sb
J16	282,83±84,77	146,01±32,54	**131,88±40,34***	232,12±106,05	Sc
J20	174,76±78,98	105,03±33,50	77,24±30,15	**32,41±22,53***	SD
J24	121,43±86,68	84,53±18,79	62,80±15,60	**7,85±10,28***	SD
J28	16,74±13,05	42,55±15,98	15,54±12,4	3,28±6,56	NS

NAT : Natural wounds, Vas : wounds treated with Vaseline, CIC : wounds treated with Cicatryl Bio, HL : wounds treated with linseed oil

NS: Not significant, S: Significant (P<0.05) *

Sa: VAS *versus* NAT and versus HLSb:VAS *versus* others

sc:CIC *versus* NAT and HLSD:HL *versus* others

At D_0 , all wounds have a comparable diameter and the same signs of inflammation. Generally, there was a progressive reduction in wound area during treatment in the different wounds.

To simplify the interpretation of the above table, it seems preferable to present the scarring process according to a given chronology.

D0-J8: "Inflammatory phase

During the first week, the smallest average surface area was recorded in wounds treated with Vaseline ($254.58±50.66cm^2$), followed by those treated with Cicatryl-Bio® ($255.66±60.54cm$).^{2}

Mean surface areas of ($347.63±77.91cm^2$) and ($418.12±127.41cm^2$) are noted in wounds treated with *Linum usitatissimum* oil and in natural (untreated) wounds respectively.

Inflammation is established as the wound surfaces initially increased in the first few days, only then did wound contraction really begin. The resorption of the inflammatory exudate started and ended in detersion, the timing of which varied with each treatment.

D8- D12: "Contraction phase

During this phase, the surface area of wounds treated with Vaseline ($211.64±20.68cm^2$) is smaller than those recorded during treatment with Cicatryl-

Bio® (237.35±50.88 cm^2) and *Linum usitatissimum* oil (320.36±34.15 cm^2). The largest average surface area was found in the natural wounds (382.35±118.18cm^2), whose contraction phase started slightly slower than the others. This confirms the overlapping phases of the healing process.

Statistically, there was a significant difference between the areas of wounds treated with Vaseline (P<0.05) and the other areas of wounds.

D_{12}- D_{16}: "Epithelialization phase

In this phase, the average surface area of wounds treated with Cicatryl-Bio® was the smallest (131.88±40.34 cm^2), with a significant difference between natural and oil-treated surfaces. The next largest difference was that of Vaseline (146.01±32.54 cm^2), both of which apparently facilitated wound hydration, thus representing the most effective products in this phase.

This was followed by the area of wounds treated with LH (232.12±106.05 cm^2), followed by those healing without treatment (282.83±84.77 cm).^{2}

D_{16}-J_{28}: "Maturation phase

After the second week, the reduction in the surface area of wounds treated with linseed oil (7.85±10.28cm^2) is faster than that of the other wounds, since statistically the oil shows its significant effect on D_{20} and D_{24}, compared to Cicatryl-Bio® (62.80±15.60cm^2), Vaseline (84.53±18.79cm^2) and the natural oil (121.43±86.68cm).^{2}

Maturation was late at D_{28} since the surfaces were still at (15.54±12.4cm2), (42.55±15.98cm^2), (16.74±13.05cm^2 ·) for wounds treated with Cicatryl-Bio® and vaseline and those not treated respectively. In contrast, the oil-treated wounds (3.28±6.56 cm^2) showed better maturation.

This illustrates the early effect of *Linum usitatissimum L* oil on epithelial regeneration of second degree burns.

The healing time is significantly faster (p<0.05) in the tested HL (26.00 ± 5.89D), compared to the different controls; similarly, CIC-treated wounds (32.50±2.87) heal before VAS-treated (35.60±3.90) and NAT-treated wounds (35.00 ± 1.16) respectively; the healing achieved by these wounds is quite comparable (see table below)

Table VI: Wound healing time **(J)**

	NAT	VAS	CIC
Mys±SD	35±1,16	35,6±3,9	32,5±2,87
HL vs.	S	S	S

26±5,89
Mys±SD:Mean± Standard deviation
HL vs: oil *vs*

2.1.2. Wound contraction

There is a progressive contraction of the wound surface from the first week (inflammatory period) in the different wounds (except for the untreated one which started to shrink in the second week).

The percentage of contraction was better in the VAS wounds (D8, and D12) but at D16, the CIC wounds statistically corrected the wound reduction with a significant effect. After this day the two products remained statistically close, with no significant difference (Table VII, Figure 14).

Statistically, the highest rate of contraction (D20 and D24) is obtained in wounds treated with HL (P<0.05) followed by CIC.

In contrast, the contraction of VAS-treated wounds is better than that of NAT wounds with no significant effect (Figure 15).

At D28, statistically, there was no significant effect *versus* the test and/or control products, maturation was completed at the same rate. Oil showed a (99%) reduction ratio, followed by CIC and NAT (95%), ending at (86%) for VAS.

Table VII: Rate (%) of wound contraction at separate intervals

	J4	J8	J12	J16	J20	J24	J28
NAT	-25,7± 26,36	-33,16± 40,46	-21,75± 37,76	10,00± 27,35	44,5 ± 25,09	61,5± 27,5	94,75± 4,35
VAS	-10,25± 4,60	19,24± 2,8	32,60± 8,60	53,5± 20,96	66,55± 14,69	73,08± 23,6	86,45± 13,67
CIC	-4,25± 2,7	18,58± 1,61	24,41± 1,75	58± 0,69	75,4± 1,96	80± 2,11	95± 10,98
HL	-6,25± 6,70	-10,75± 24,58	-02,02± 10,86	26,07± 33,78	90 ± 06,98	97,50± 03,32	99,0± 02
P	NS	S	S	S	S	S	NS
Variant	-	VAS/NAT VAS /HL	VAS/Other	CIC/NAT CIC /HL	HL /Other	HL /Other	-

NS: Not significant
S: Significant (P<0.05)

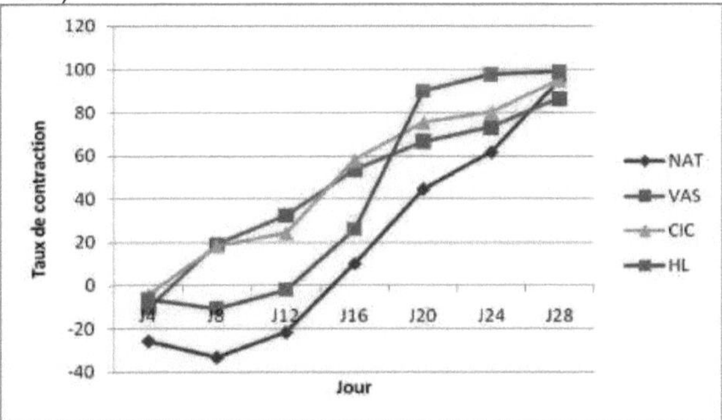

Figure 14: Evolution of wound contraction

The photos below show the shrinkage of the different wounds as a function of the duration of treatment (figure 14).

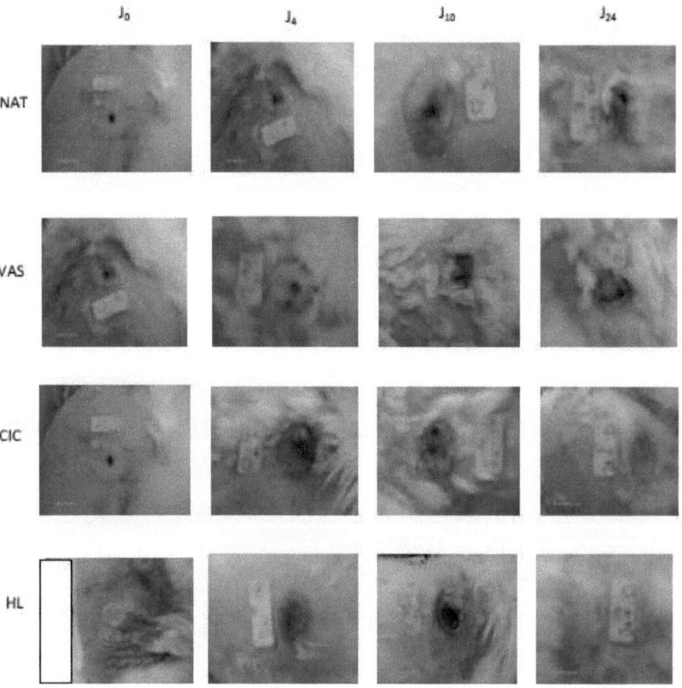

Figure 15: Chronology of wound healing

2.2. Clinical study

2.2.1. General condition

During the test period, no deaths were observed in the rabbits, all animals remained healthy and available to evaluate the efficacy of linseed oil in healing burns.

2.2.2. Overweight status

The mean weight of the rabbits did not change significantly ($p>0.05$) from the initial mean weight (3411.25± 325.38g). The weights obtained after burns varied slightly: (3401±329.93g) at D_7 , (3426.25±351.50g) at D_{14} , (3452.5±351.41g) at D_{21}, (3432.5±351.67g) at D_{28} and (3470±352.30g) at D_{35} (Table VIII, figure 16).

The daily application of the test products did not significantly alter the body development of the rabbits. The weight gain obtained after 35 days of application was 1.7% (3470.5±352.30g), expressing the conditions of the animal house during the different stages of the procedure and the age and growth achieved by the rabbits.

Table VIII: Average weight (g) of rabbits burnt at different intervals

Days	J_0	J7	J_{14}	J_{21}	J_{28}	J_{35}
Weight means±	3411,25±	3401±	3426,25±	3452,5±	3432,5±	3470±
Standard deviation	325,38	329,93	351,50	351,41	351,67	352,30

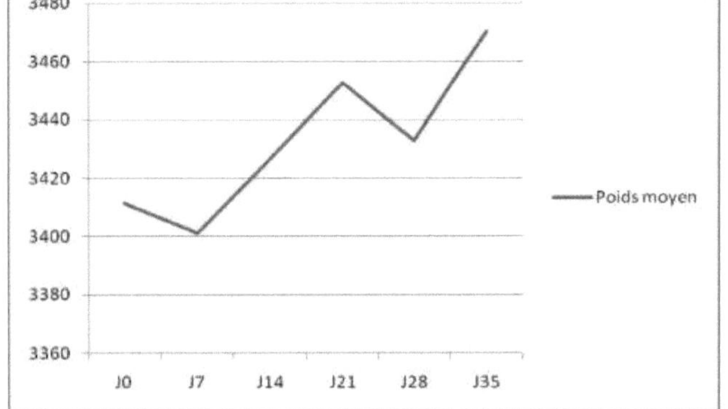

Figure 16: Evolution of the average body weight of burnt rabbits

2.3. Histological study

Histological examination shows that the wounds (natural, Vaseline and Cicatryl-Bio treated) show destruction of an area of the epidermis, subepidermal bullous lesion (epidermal detachment) and the presence of increased fibrosis with infiltration by chronic inflammatory elements, which seems to be responsible for delayed healing (Figure 17 A-C).

In contrast, wounds treated with linseed oil show thinning of the epidermis, the appearance of a discrete fibrosis of the superficial dermis which is relatively reworked, a sub-epidermal layer infiltrated with a few dispersed mono-nucleated inflammatory elements and more marked neo-vascularisation of the granulation tissue, favouring a good quality scar (figure 16D).

Finally, histological examination shows that the inflammatory phase is almost complete and the reparative phase is well established in the wounds treated with linseed oil, whereas the other wounds show significant fibrosis, persistent inflammatory infiltration and a distinctly less developed tissue repair phase.

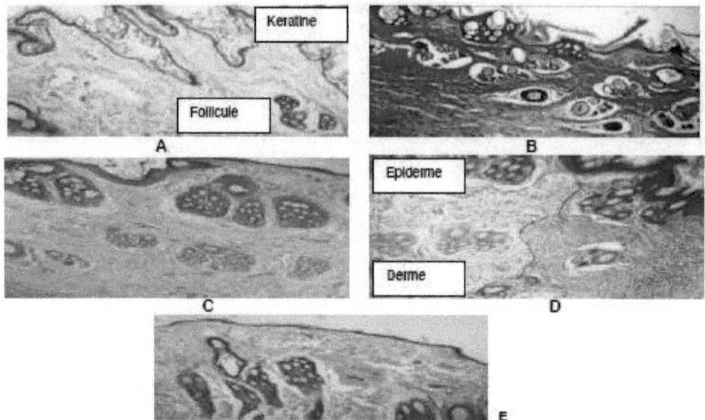

Figure 17: Microphotographs of histological sections of the skin (HE X10)
A: Natural burn, **B:** Burn treated with Vaseline, **C:** Burn treated with Cicatryl-Bio,
D : Burn treated with linseed oil. **E** : Healthy skin

3. DISCUSSION

3.1. Wound planimetry

From a clinical point of view, *Linum usitatissimum* oil favours the inflammatory phase because at D4, the surface area of the wounds treated with the oil increased by 6% compared to the initial surface area and by 10% at D_8 . This is in agreement with the results of Park and Barbul (2004) who report that the 6 days following the burns correspond to the inflammatory phase (erythema and redeme).

The results obtained are different from Kabarinta (2010) who observed 30 and 34% wound shrinkage on D5 using *Opilia celtidifolia* leaf ointments and those of Djerrou et al (2013b) and Maameri (2014) who reported that lentisk oil improved the healing effect on D4 (36-33% wound surface contraction).

The highest rate is reported in the study by Suntar et al (2011), 56.5% contraction of incision and excision wounds (rats and mice) at D6, treated with methanolic extract *of Rubus sanctusa*.

Statistically, there was a significant difference between the areas of the study wounds treated with Vaseline and the other wounds (P<0.05).

Vaseline treatment showed good inflammation compared to the other products tested. Indeed, Pu et al (1999), mention that in the early stage of the healing process, petroleum jelly is able to inhibit the evaporation of water from the wound. Thus, it is known that a moist physiological environment must be formed in the wound for skin repair and regeneration of damaged tissue. However, prolonged therapy can lead to tissue damage and maceration (Xu and Xiao, 2003).

The process of progressive contraction started late from D12 with the appearance of a crust on the surface; presumably inflammation overcame the contraction of the linseed oil treated wounds. This is in agreement with the findings of Fournier and Mordon (2005), who report that the different phases of wound healing overlap and that one phase cannot be fully completed without the second phase progressively setting in simultaneously.

In contrast, Djerrou et al, (2010) and Maameri et al, (2012) observe that contraction starts in the first week. In contrast to the data of Kabarinta (2010) who observed complete wound healing between 11 and 17 days. Shanmuga Priya et al (2002) report complete wound closure within 12 days in rats treated with *Datura alba* extract. From D16 onwards, contraction resumed instantaneously, following the detachment of the crust. This period is characterised by the formation of granulation tissue and epithelialisation (Martin, 1997; Singer and Clark, 1999; MacKay and Miller, 2003; Enoch and Leaper, 2005 in Belfadel, 2009). It corresponds to half of the second proliferative and remodelling phase (Park and Barbul, 2004).

The contraction rate of wounds treated with linseed oil is 26%. Maameri (2014) reports higher contraction rates using mastic oil alone (76%) and a mixture of mastic oil with honey (70%). Thus, the traditional ointment (pine gum, onion, mugwort, beeswax and fresh butter) was superior. It showed a 93% reduction in surface area at D15, which is probably explained by the rapidity of wound healing in laboratory rats and particularly by the efficiency of the legendary formula well known in the Constantine region (eastern Algeria) (Bensegueni et al, (2007). Boulebda et al, (2009), note that the contraction of wounds treated with mastic oil is 92% at D18 after the incision of the skin of rats. The ethanol extract of *Zyziphus oenoplia* gave a distinct wound shrinkage of 97% close to that of the positive control (Framycetin) at D16 (Majunder, 2010). *Teucrium polium gave* a contraction of (96-97%) at D15, on excision wounds (Boutaleb, 2014)

The wound contraction rates (at D15) for Madecassol and Vaseline are 72.27% and 71.2% respectively (Sifour et al, 2012). In addition, our wound contraction rates are lower; 58% of burns treated with Cicatryl Bio and 53% with Vaseline.

Low rates are recorded after treatment of wounds between D20 and D24 with Cicatryl Bio® (75% and 80%), with Vaseline (66% and 73%) and in those not treated (44% and 61%).

The use of linseed oil allowed a better reduction of the surface area during epithelialization (90% and 97%) between D_{20} and D_{24} ; this is in agreement with the results of Aouina and Remili (2013) who report that the contraction of wounds treated with *Lepidium sativum* is 90% at D23 (burns experimented on rabbits). In contrast to the results of Djerrou (2011), who reported a reduction rate of 88% in wounds treated with mastic oil at D24.

The active contraction of the wound surface treated with linseed oil is 99% at D28. This result is close to that reported by Djerrou (2014), who tested a mixture of *Fagopyrum Esculentum* with honey and observed a contraction rate of 99% at D27. In contrast, after D26, wound contraction was complete (100%) in rats treated with mastic oil (Belfadel, 2009).

Our work shows that the maturation time of the burns is in the range of 21-26 days. This is in agreement with the results obtained by Hamdi Pacha et al, (2002) on several plants: *Juneperus Oxycedrus*, *Pinus Alepensis* (23-25 days), *Lawsonia Inermis* and *Cedrus Atlantica* (17-20 days) but slightly lower than that of *Inula Viscosa* (28 days).

Compared to our results, Srivastava and Durgaprasad (2008) reported a long epithelialization time of 39 days for the *Cocos nucifera* oil-treated group of rats. Djerrou (2011) and Djerrou et al (2013b) found slow maturation at D30, although the contraction of mastic oil-treated burns was very early but with a gradual and rather prolonged rhythm.

Furthermore, Benlaksira et al, (2013) showed that the mixture of juice and *Opuntia ficus indica* seed gives a short time to healing with a maturation of 20-21 days. In addition, these same authors noted a maturation time quite close (21-24D) to that obtained (21-26 days) when testing the juice extract of the cactus seed.

In the literature, most studies have evaluated the healing activity of topical application of some plants.

Singularly, *Cinnamomum zeylanicum* bark extract is administered orally at a dose of 250mg/kg and 500mg/kg body weight.

The rate of wound contraction and the period of epithelialisation in excisional wounds is better than in the control (Kamath et al, 2003).

Linseed oil showed a better healing effect compared to the products tested. Indeed, this oil gave on the one hand, a rather prolonged period of inflammation and on the other hand, a 90% retraction from D20. Statistically a significant difference *to* other products tested was observed. Very high rates were observed until complete healing (D_{28}), with no sign of infection.

The properties of the components of the plant oil, *Linum usitatissimum L,* could justify its action during the phases of the epithelial regeneration process and thus explain its healing effect.

Numerous studies have shown that plants traditionally used as healing agents have immune system activating properties; this activation is thought to be the mechanism of wound healing. Flaxseed protein is an excellent source of arginine, glutamine and histidine. These three amino acids are known to stimulate the immune system (Oomah, 2001).

Other studies have also shown that polysaccharides are substances responsible for the activation of the immune system and thus for wound healing (Yamada and Kiyohara 1999; Nergard 2005). The presence of polysaccharides in flax is reported by Rubilar et al (2010)

Flaxseed oil (*Linum usitatissimum*) is one of the richest sources of n-3 fatty acids (FA) in the plant world. Among the wide range of activities, omega-3s have a great impact on skin physiology (Maurette, 2008) and its healing activity (Derek et al, 1999; McDaniel et al, 2008)

Linoleic acid and alpha-linoleic acid provide lipids necessary for cell membrane repair and cell respiration (Loden and Andersson, 1996). In general, fatty acids and triglycerides are able to reduce trans epidermal water loss and thus increase skin hydration. It has been shown that healing plants often have a high level of plant sterols (Dweck, 2002).

There are reports that vitamin E increases the rate of healing and improves the aesthetic outcome of burns, as alpha-tocopherol has a powerful antioxidant action (Palmeri et al, 1995; Martin, 1996; Baumann and Spencer, 1999). Flax also contains lignins which belong to the phytoestrogen family; these lignins have anti-oxidant and anti-cancer properties (Prasad, 1997; Prasad, 2000; Chen et al, 2002; Thompson, 2003; Zanwar et al, 2010).

Flaxseed oil has antimicrobial activity against *Staphylococcus aureus, Streptococcus agalactiae, Enterococcus faecalis, Micrococcus luteus, Bacillus subtilis and Candida albicans* (Kaithwas et al, 2011). This would explain the good epithelial regeneration in the absence of infection in treated wounds.

3.2. Evolution of body weight

The daily application of the different products tested did not disturb the general condition of the rabbits, no mortality and/or clinical signs were found. The body evolution of the rabbits did not show any significant difference, which is consistent with the work of Aouina and Remili (2013) and Maameri (2014). The latter used at the beginning of the experiment rabbits weighing 2500 g, whereas in this study the average weight of the rabbits is 3500 g. This difference in weight could explain the difference between the average gains recorded which is probably due to the physiological acquisition of the adult weight of the selected rabbits (3500g) at 10 months. A slight slowdown in weight growth of the study animals was observed in the first week, followed by a resumption of weight growth until the end of the experiment. These results clearly show that the decrease in body weight irrespective of the nature of the treatment is probably related to the direct effect of the lesion trauma and other pathophysiological factors in the wound healing process (Belfadel, 2009).

3.3. Histological observation

The inflammatory phase is almost complete and the repair phase is well established in the burns treated with *Linum usitatissimum* oil.

This result is comparable to that reported by various authors who have conducted experiments on rats:

- Dense collagen, fewer macrophages and good capillary formation after wound treatment with *Zyziphus oenoplia* extract (Majunder (2010).

- On day 28, wounds treated with *Cramoll* hydrogel showed complete epithelialisation of the tissue. On day 35eme , dense collagenous tissue is observed (Dos Tavares Pereira et al, 2012).

- The data observed by Bouteleb (2014), reveal that neo-vascularisation is more marked at D_{12}, in wounds treated with *Teucrium polium.*

- In the histo-pathological study by Shivare et al (2014b), new blood vessels, fibroblast cells and collagen fibres are found in the group treated with *Trichosanthes dioica* extract.

In contrast, the other wounds (NAT, VAS) in the present study show significant fibrosis, inflammatory infiltration and a distinctly less advanced phase of tissue repair, similar to the following work:

- Bensegueni (2007) observed a barely rough epithelium (less mature granulation tissue) in untreated (control) burns at D_{15} . Concerning the importance of the exudate evoked by the same author and compared with the burns treated with ointment. In our study, the wounds do not show the pathophysiological action of leucogenes.

- Thus Majunder (2010) reports the importance of macrophages and fibroblasts and less vascularisation and collagen in the control group section.

- At D_2, an inflammatory infiltrate (leukocytes) is observed in each group while at D_7, each group had evidence of fibroblast proliferation.

Groups treated with *Copaifera langsdorffli oleoresin* showed fewer fibroblasts and more organised collagen fibres at J_{14} compared to saline (Masson Meyers et al, 2013).

It is recalled **that** the evaluation of the healing activity of linseed oil (*Linum usitatissimum L*) is assessed following experimental burns in laboratory rabbits. The healing process went through several phases: a gradual disappearance of inflammation (wounds became less red and less voluminous), a contraction phase (wounds became hard and covered with slightly black crusts); the treatment made it possible to obtain a complete healing of the wounds. According to the results obtained, it appears that:

• *Linum usitatissimum* is tolerable, causing no inflammation or irritation to the healthy skin surrounding the wounds.

• From a planimetric point of view, this oil promotes the inflammatory phase gradually, which is essential for the healing process. It stimulates contraction, reducing the surface area of wounds during the epithelialisation phase. The difference became significant compared to other wounds; at 20eme day (90%), and at 24eme day (97%).

• This oil does not have a negative effect on the healing process, no clinical disturbance has been observed.

• Histologically, in the wounds treated with oil, an attenuation of inflammation and an increase in granulation tissue are noted, which attests to good epithelial regeneration.

Finally, a positive effect of *Linum usitatissimum* oil during the healing process of second-degree burns in adult rabbits is noted.

CHAPTER VI : ESTIMATION OF HAIR REGROWTH (OIL AND SEED)

Although hair loss (alopecia) is not a disabling or fatal disease, the very thought of going bald can lead to emotional stress. Suitably effective medications are available, however, and many are wary of their unknown long-term effects and possible side effects. This leads to increased interest in alternative remedies. Preclinical trials of good scientific quality on plants are possible but rarely elaborated (Guedje et al, 2012).

Among the plants used in traditional medicine, *Linum usitatissimum* has the reputation of being efficient.

To determine the effect of the plant (seed and its pure oil) on hair growth (hair system), the oil is tested by external application (Test B: topical) and the ground seed by digestion (Test C1: gavage). The two tests are performed separately on rabbits ranging from 6 to 12 in number. Using the same procedure, the dimensions of a head are measured, i.e. the length, the diameter of the plucked hairs and the weight of the shaved hairs.

1. **MATERIALS** (Annex 9)

2. **METHODS**

2.1. Distribution of lots

For the purpose of this section, two tests are set up (figure 14), according to the two forms of presentation of the plant (oil+seed) (tests: B+C1) with four (04) batches of comparable rabbits. Two batches of rabbits were used for each test. The animal material was subjected to the same environmental, temperature and hygiene conditions as described above.

2.2. Topical application

For the realization of the first test: B: "external application of the oil", whose duration of measurement is 04 weeks, the twelve (12) rabbits are divided into 02 batches:

An *oil* batch: daily, linseed oil ($1ml/100cm^2$) is applied to the delimited surface of the shaved back of each rabbit. At the same time, another batch of **Natural** was used for comparison of natural regrowth without any treatment, on the surface under consideration. A straitjacket is placed immediately after application of the products for 10 minutes, to prevent immediate licking (figure 18Ab).

2.3. Digestive supplementation

For the execution of the second test: C1 "seed ingestion", with a trial period of 18 successive weeks, the first of which is an adaptation week, this test required the constitution of two batches of 12 rabbits for each:

-In the Seed lot, each subject is fed daily with ground flaxseed (Figure 18Bc) for 13 weeks at the dose (1g/kg/day), another comparable lot (*Control)* is fed with an empty syringe, without any feed supplement (these same lots were used to explore the safety of the seed; Test C2). The rabbits are restrained with a towel (Figure 18Bb)

At week 13, six rabbits from each batch were sacrificed; the remaining six were kept to contribute to and control the effect of the seed after one month of deprivation, they were abruptly stopped from ingesting the seed, without any supplementation for another 4 successive weeks (*Cinetic* batch).

2.4. How it works

The criteria controlled for the quantitative evaluation of hair growth (Test: B, and C1) are the parameters of fleece production, i.e. length, width and weight of the hair collected (Rougeaut and Thebault, 1983; Rochambeau and Vrillon, 1985).

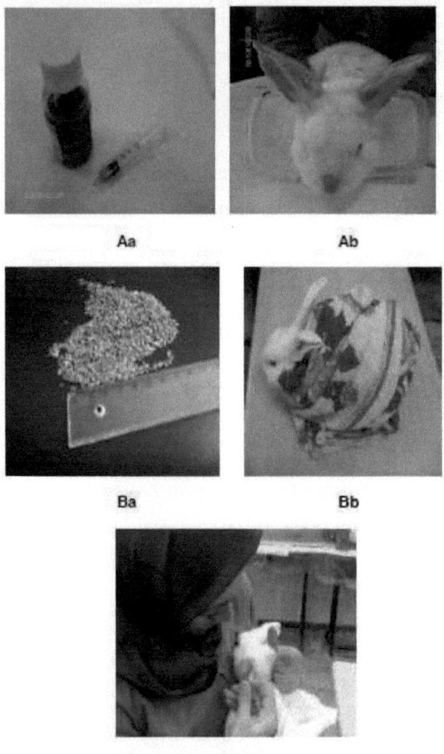

Figure 18: Two experimental routes of flax administration
Aa: Linseed oil, **Ab**: Carcan in place
Ba: Whole flaxseed, **Bb**: Rabbit restraint, **Bc**: Rabbit feeding

The study was conducted according to the technique described by Thebault (1977) and slightly modified by Purwal, et al (2008).

1. A bunch of hair is removed by tweezers immediately before each shave on the rabbit's back.

2. A surface shave is performed once a month (04 weeks) (figure19:A-B)

3. A template is used to mark out a square area (10x10cm) on the back of each animal for all batches (Figure 19C).

4. The dimensions of a dozen hairs (one sample) are measured (length and diameter) using a graduated ruler and a microscope with a micrometer on the objective (zoom) 10 respectively.

The length is measured by simply reading the scale placed on the blade by pulling on the hair, these measurements are made to the nearest millimetre, only on the "body" of the hair excluding the bulging parts of the "heads".

5. The shaved surface hair is weighed using a high precision balance (KERN plus, Max=510, d=0.001g) and stored in a labelled bag specific to each rabbit (Figure 19D).

6. A session of boundary photography is taken weekly on the back of each rabbit in the different batches.

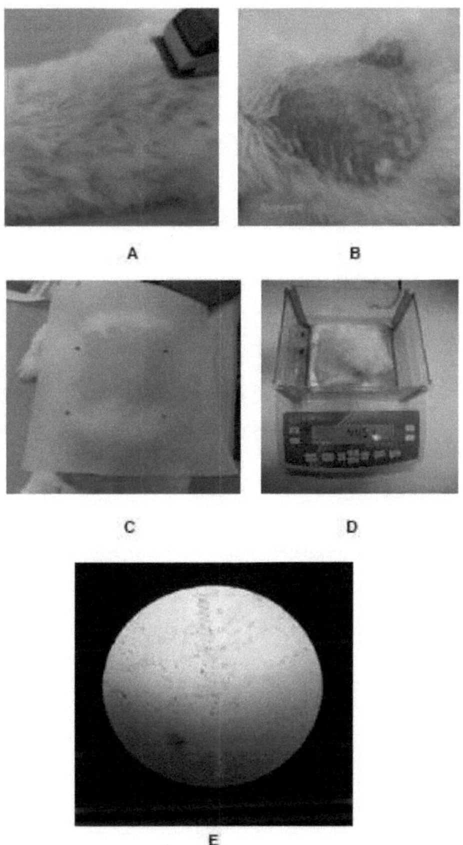

Figure 19: Different stages of hair regrowth assessment

A, B: Rabbit back shaving, **C**: Surface template, **D**: Hair weighing,

E: Micrometer microphotograph

3. RESULTS AND DISCUSSION

3.1. Test B results

The hair size results represent the mean ± standard deviation, calculated for 06 rabbits of each batch and the Matlab program gave the value of P (Table IX).

After 04 weeks of topical application, the hair length was 2.38±0.79cm, it was

2.72±0.76cm in rabbits without treatment. In contrast, the hair width of the **Oil** and **Natural** batches was 39.00±21.39pm and 27.17±15.52pm respectively. In the untreated lot, the weight of the hair collected was 0.76±0.17g, in the treated lot it was 1.17±1.66g.

The decrease is marked in the hair length (12%), in the **Oil** lot with no statistical difference, the width and the weight of the collected mass showed an increase (43% and 53% respectively) compared to the **Natural** lot.

Linseed oil improved hair width and crop weight but not length. Statistically, the hair width of the treated lot showed a slight significant difference from the **natural** lot (P < 9%).

Table IX: Hair dimensions of the two batches of test B

	Length (cm)	Width (pm)	Weight (g)
Natural	2.72±0.76	27.17±15.52	0.76±0.17
Oil	2.38±0.79	39.00±21.39	1.17±1.66
P	NS	S	NS

NS: Not significant
S: Significant

The figure below shows the evolution of body weights during the four weeks of the test. A variation is noted between the 3eme week and the 4eme week, in both test batches (Natural, Oil), without any significant difference.

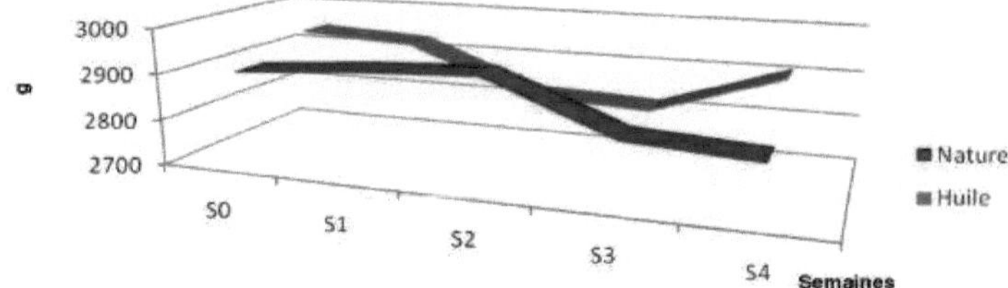

Figure 20: Evolution of body weight in test B rabbits

3.2. Discussion of Test B

Several authors have indicated that fur quality depends on factors such as sex, environment, conditions, season, photoperiodism and sampling method (shaving or hair removal) (Charlet-lery et al, 1985; Rochambeau and Vrillon, 1985).

Therefore, the rabbits used in our study are of the same sex and breed. They are kept under the same environmental conditions.

The criteria for selecting a route of administration depend on clinical, pharmacological and pathophysiological parameters and the cost of treatment. The oral route (per-os) is the most commonly used route. The drug is absorbed either in the gastric mucosa or in the intestine. It then enters the general circulation. In contrast, the cutaneous route is a local route; the drug is applied directly *in situ*. It exerts its action at the precise site of the disease. The low diffusion of the active product beyond the site of administration limits the undesirable effects (Ruckebusch, 1981; Bourin, 1991).

The dose tested and the duration of the test vary from study to study; 1ml/4cm^2 for 30 days (d'Adhrijan et al, 2003), 0.2ml/mouse for 30 days (Rho et al, 2005), 100^l/8cm^2 for 4 weeks (Harada et al, 2008), 0.2ml/mouse for three weeks (Kang-Bong et al, 2011) and 0.4ml/rat for 21 days (Upadhyay et al, 2012; Upadhyay et al, 2014).

The present study demonstrated the quantitative effect of *Linum usitatissimum* on hair growth in rabbits at a dose of 1 ml/100 cm^2 for a period of 4 weeks.

However, the daily application of the tested linseed oil did not disturb the general condition of the rabbits, no clinical and/or dermatological signs were found. The body evolution of the rabbits did not show any significant difference, which is in agreement with the work of Kang-Bong et al, (2011).

Daily oil treatment shows an increase in hair width and density (weight/area) after 4 weeks of topical application.

Statistically, the hair width of the oil-treated batch increased by a small significant difference *compared to* the natural batch. The increase in hair density was more than 50% without significant effect.

Furthermore, linseed oil provides a certain stimulus to the hair system, the mechanism of action of which is not yet established and remains a promising support to be confirmed by future work.

The study by Adhrijan et al (2003) reported that *Hibiscus rosa-sinensis* leaf extract had a strong effect on albino rat hair growth compared to flower extract. The increase in hair length was 25% compared to the control group.

Prunus dulcis extraction showed a consistent and significant increase in the length of albino rat hair and hair follicle in the anagen phase after histological studies. The time required to complete hair growth is 24 days (Suraj et al, 2009).

Also, *Zizyphus jujuba* essential oil is applied at different concentrations to the skin of the shaved back of mice for 21 days.

Hair weight is higher (14%) for mice treated with the plant (Yoon et al, 2010).

Thus *Glycyrrhiza glabra* extract gave an increase in hair length (36%) compared to the control group (Upadhyay et al, 2012 b).

In general, the tested extracts showed a considerable hair length activity comparable to that of the standard drug "Minoxidil", paradoxically to the effect of *Linum usitatissimum* oil, the hair width showed a significant difference at D_{28}.

It is likely that the effect of promoting hair growth is due to hormonal stimulation of the plant extract. Restrogens prolong the anagen phase of hair growth, whereas androgens are responsible for hair loss (Upadhyay et al, 2012 a,b).

It should be remembered that the behaviour of lignans (polyphenolic compounds) depends on the biological level of restradiol. At physiological restradiol levels, lignans act as restrogen antagonists, but in menopausal women (low restradiol levels), they cause a decrease in restrogen (Rickard and Thompson, 1997; Hutchins and Slavin, 2003). In addition, flax is the richest cereal in lignan secoisolariciresinol diglycoside (SDG) (Patterson, 2006), which may have an effect on hair growth.

A number of researchers have shown that flavonoids have an activity on hair growth by strengthening the capillary wall of small blood vessels supplying the hair follicles; these components improve blood circulation thus promoting hair growth (Kobayashi et al, 1993). Others also involve flavonoids to stimulate the transformation of the telogen phase into anagen. They also induce the expression of certain growth factors, such as growth insulin-like factor-1 (IGF-1), vascular endothelial growth factors (VEGF), keratinocyte growth factors (KGF) and hepatocyte growth factors (HGF), all of which have stimulatory effects on hair follicle growth (Tomoya et al, 1999; Roh et al, 2002; Roh et al, 2005).

3.3. C1 test results

The observed data from the seed supplementation are statistically studied, tabulated and interpreted as they are obtained. Two sick rabbits are excluded from the interpretation of the results.

3.3.1. Length of the teeth

The results obtained (Table X and Figure 21) do not show a significant variation in length between the control and seed lots (P>0.05).

Nevertheless, from S_{04} to S_{12}, increases of 34% and 26% are observed for the control and seed lots respectively. Lower growth rates of 3.5% (control) and 7.3% (seed) are observed from S_0 to S_{12}. A time effect (P=0.006) was revealed at 8eme weeks compared to 4eme in the seed lot.

Table X: Average length (cm) of axe

	S_0	S_4	S_8	S_{12}	S_{16}
Witness	2.240±0.940	1.737±0.689	2.692±0.606	2.325±1.026	2.72±0.76
Seed	1.900±0.881	1.655±0.735	*2.080±0.618	2.043±1.233	2.25±0.53
Regime effect	-	NS	NS	NS	NS

NS: Not significant
* Significant (P<0.01)

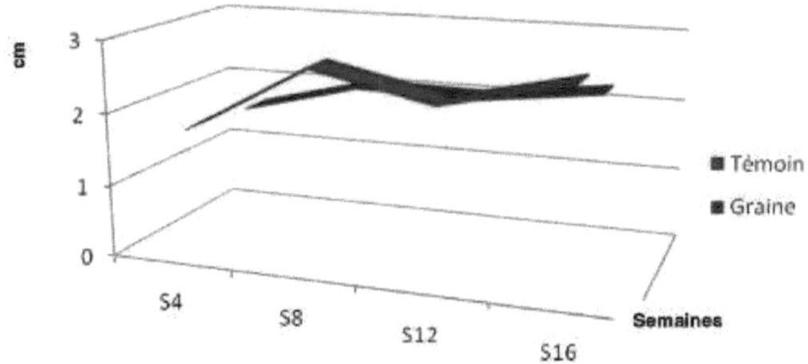

Figure 21: Average length (cm) of axe

3.3.2. Width of treads

Table XI shows the average width (um) of the sampled logs. It can be seen that the width decreased in both batches. However, a slightly significant increase (7%) was observed at S_{12} (P=0.09) in the seed lot *versus the* control lot.

Upon withdrawal (s16) of the supplementation for 4 weeks, a decrease (5.6%) in hair width was again observed in the cinetic lot at the 5[eme] hair harvest compared to the 4[eme] harvest (seed lot at s12) (Figure 22). In contrast, a highly significant widening (40%) in the cinetic lot was obtained compared to the control lot (P=0.006).

Table XI: Average width (um) of millstones

	So	S4	S8	S12	S16
Witness	50.00±24.36	48.00±32.61	45.50±17.60	32.58±19.67	27.17±15.52
Seed	54.88±27.74	50.88±28.02	37.61±25.69	40.25±22.10	38.00±17.10

Effect

-NSNSSS

regime
NS: Not significant
S: Significant

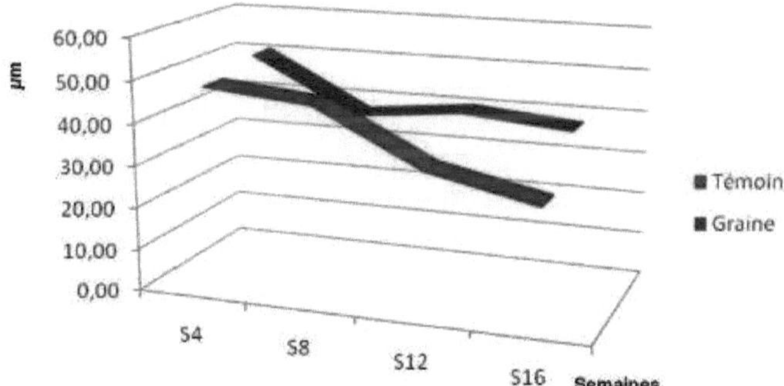

Figure 22 : Evolution de la largeur des mèches

3.3.3. Hair weighing

The shaved areas (108) show variances in hair mass in both batches over the three months. However, flaxseed ingestion showed a highly significant effect (P=0.02) on

79

hair weight (density) at 3eme harvest (S_8) compared to 2eme. This effect disappeared immediately afterwards (Table XII).

After 12 weeks of ingestion, hair weighing showed no beneficial effect of flaxseed compared to the control lot. Similarly, the average weight showed a sharp decrease which continued after 4 weeks of supplementation was withdrawn (figure 23).

Table XII: Average weight (g) of hair collected

	So	S4	S_8	S_{12}	S16
Witness	3.89±1.43	1.24±0.87	2.04±1.89	0.46±0.47	0.76±0.17
Seed	3.92±0.80	0.53±0.53	*1.47±0.77	0.88±0.92	0.24±0.16
Regime effect	-	NS	NS	NS	NS

NS: Not significant
* Significant (P<0.05)

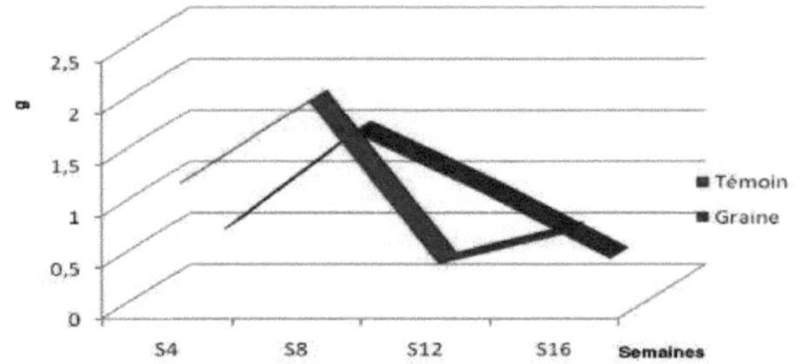

Figure 23: Evolution of the weight of the cheeses.

3.3.4. Evaluation of the two tests

The results of the two routes of administration (test: B, 4 weeks of topical application of 1ml flaxseed oil daily and test: C1, 12 weeks of daily dietary supplementation of the seed) are shown in Table XIII).

The distinction is notable, given the specificity and particularity of each of the two routes (dermal and oral), they are unquestionably different.

However, as an indication, oil application was significantly (P=0.04) more effective in increasing hair length *than* seed ingestion. Thus, a decrease (6%) in hair width and an increase (30%) in weight were recorded, compared to the seed lot, but without significant effect.

Therefore, ingestion of flaxseed has a slight beneficial effect on hair width after 12 weeks of supplementation, which is more interesting in 4 weeks with topical application of flaxseed oil compared to the natural batch.

Compared to the seed lot, some improvement in hair length (18%), a decrease in width (8%) and a drop in weight (70%) were observed in the Cinetic lot, without any significant difference.

Table XIII: Estimated parameters of the two routes of administration

	Length (cm)	Width (pm)	Weight (g)
Oil	2.38±0.79	39.00±21.39	1.17±1.66
Seed	1.90±0.51	41.33±24.60	0.82±1.16
Cinetics	2.25±0.53	38.00±17.10	0.24±0.16

3.4. Discussion of the C1 test

A variability in the dimensions (length and width) of the hairs measured during the test is observed, which ensures at least that the ingestion of the seed does not block the hair system in its physiological cycle, but it stimulates it slightly since there is a positive effect on the width and a satisfactory reinforcement of the length of the hairs from the second month on.

Thibaut (1977) confirms that the rate of hair growth is different as it increases rapidly between the 6th and 7th week after hair removal and becomes specific and unique to each hair category between the 9th and 13th week. Thus the length diagram agrees that 2-3% of the lengths are superior to the others and do not belong to the same tylotrich population.

This coincides with the fluctuations observed in the present study, where the harvest is carried out every four weeks just before the increase and the specificity of the physiological hair growth.

Hair removal induces the synchronous growth of a new, perfectly structured coat, but following shearing, the coat normally continues to grow with a proportion of hairs cut off, leading to a fleece lacking in structure (Rougeot and Thebault, 1983). This can probably justify the decrease in width and weight recorded in the control lot, as the harvest progresses from 2eme to 5eme .

Similarly, the quantitative evolution of hair obtained is fluctuating, it agrees with the bibliographic synthesis carried out by Bernard (2006) who confirms that the hair follicle is the only stable cutaneous appendage by its asynchronous and stochastic cyclicity.

The transformation of hair follicles from the telogen to the anagen phase in the treated groups could be due to the proliferation of epithelial cells at the base of the follicles inducing vasodilation of blood vessels in the scalp (Uno and Kurata (1993); Savin and Atton (1993); Jain et al, 2006). Histological studies have shown a clear increase in follicle size during the active phase and a concomitant increase in the vascular bed around the follicles (Thorburn et al, 2012).

At the same time, the development of the vascular network allows the supply of all the nutrients that the hair needs for its growth. The latter is ensured by the multiplication of the root's generative cells (Clere, 2010). Indeed, it is known that the chemical components of flax play the role of antioxidant, anti-cancer and anti-estrogenic. They stabilise DNA during cell division (Oomah, 2001; Patterson, 2006).

In addition, hair growth is inhibited by the administration of paracrine growth factors such as EGF (epithelial growth factor) (Tsuboi, 1997). The latter is inhibited by the use of linseed (Tan et al, 2004). Thus, ALA (alpha-linoleic acid) in flaxseed oil can help inhibit 5 alpha reductase type 2, the enzyme responsible for the conversion of testosterone to dihydrotestosterone (DHT). This male hormone shrinks hair follicles and alters the cyclic phase of a hair growth cycle (Li, 1992; Liang and Liao 1997; Galcera, 2002; Brenner, 2003). In addition, flax is the best source of alpha linoleic acid (Oomah, 2001).

In addition, chutney flaxseed regime has been shown to stimulate the level of y-glutamyl transpeptidase (Faseehuddin and Basavaraj, 2007). This microsomal enzyme is an indicator of hair growth (together with alkaline phosphatase) (Kang-Bong et al, 2011).

All these studies could explain the beneficial effect observed in the flaxseed ingestion test.

Although the origin of hair loss has not been elucidated, it is characterised by a progressive increase in the heterogeneity of hair diameter and by the appearance of peripilary signs, the signature of a temporary inflammatory phase that seems to precede the thickening of the connective sheath and the miniaturisation of the follicle (Deloche et al, 2004).

In parallel, an increase in hair width is mainly obtained with topical application of linseed oil for 4 weeks. The latter is also noted after 13 weeks of daily flaxseed ingestion. It ensures a continuous effect for another four weeks after withdrawal of the supplement. During this time, the oil confirms its interest by its convenience, its duration of administration and the absence of any dermatological damage.

3.5. Objective limits

The present study shows a lack of apparatus for sorting hairs (jars, beards, down), histological sectioning of the skin separating hair follicles into anagen, catagen and telogen phases.

There is also a deficiency in the micrometer calibration slide to discuss the recorded dimensions. These limitations are one of the issues that need to be addressed to ensure the results of future *in vivo* work.

To summarise, topical application of linseed oil results in a marked decrease in hair length (12%), an increase in width (43%) and in the weight of the harvested mass

(53%).

The use of this oil may be a promising treatment for alopecia and baldness, but further trials are needed to evaluate its effects on the number of hair follicles in the skin, the structure of the hair and its chemical composition. In addition, the exact mechanism of action, the plant component responsible for this activity and the appropriate dose should be studied.

It is also interesting to test linseed oil on the hair of mice and/or rats in order to know the real ranking of the plants by comparing the quantitative effect of each of them.

The results of the daily supplementation of flaxseed are original (very few studies in Algeria) in relation to the trichogenic effect since an increase in length is evaluated at the third month (26%), with a slight significant increase in the width (7%) of the hindquarters taken from the backs of the rabbits in the seed lot compared to the control.

It should be pointed out that the results obtained do not allow us to claim that the ingestion of linseed has a particular action on the morphology of the hair (structure/composition), although it does motivate the width of the hair. This result is more interesting with oil, however, a precise dosage must be determined and further studies are needed to further investigate the issue.

CHAPTER VII: TESTING FOR SEED SAFETY

The identification of new potentially active molecules is difficult, so testing the safety and efficacy of each one is a costly process. Toxicity assessment relies on the use of parameters and/or health indicators more or less specific to biological monitoring and to the association of organic lesions affecting the skin, liver and kidney (Viau and Tardif, 2003)

During the test of ingestion of ground flaxseed by daily gavage, the safety of the seed by repeated ingestion (Test: C2) is explored in parallel for three months (sub chronic toxicity). This is achieved by inserting health indicators into the experimental mode, namely clinical observation, biochemical examination and histological study of the filter organs (liver, kidneys) for the two batches of rabbits (*Seed* and *Control*)

1. **MATERIALS:** (Annex 10)

2. **METHODS**

2.1. Protocol

The steps of the investigation protocol (Figure 24), concerning the safety (Test C2) of the seed are as follows:

1. Before feeding the animals, careful observation is made on the individual sheet of the animal's behaviour, height, condition of the feed troughs and appearance of the faeces.

2. Each week, the weight of the rabbits is taken (on the same day, at the same time of day, just before feeding) (figure 24A). It is recorded on an individual card (Appendix 6).

3. Each month, a blood sample is taken from the medial marginal vein for both batches (Figure 24B).

4. At the end of the test, in the third month (M_3), the rabbits are sacrificed, after skinning and evisceration, a sample of liver and kidney tissue is taken and stored in labelled formalin bottles for subsequent histological study (Figure 24C).

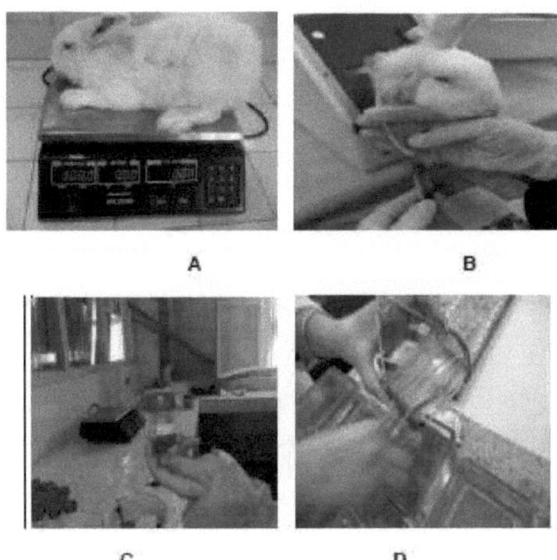

Figure 24: Different stages of safety monitoring

A: Weight gain, **B**: Blood sample, **C**: Preservation of organ samples,
D: Slide in alcohol for histological examination

2.2. Blood sampling

Blood sampling from the marginal ear vein is commonly used. It is necessary to apply a local anaesthetic cream for 20-30 min prior to bleeding which helps prevent the animal from shaking its head. The needle is pushed through the skin, 2.5-3ml of blood is collected in a heparin tube.

The vein should be compressed for at least 2 minutes to prevent further bleeding and hematoma. The animal should be checked for persistent bleeding 5 and 10 minutes later.

The heparin tubes are centrifuged (Hettich zentrifugen EBA 20) at 3000 rpm for 5 minutes, the collected plasma is dispensed into two dry labelled tubes and stored at -18°C, until use.

2.3. Biochemical assay

The selected blood parameters are performed by an automatic analyser (Architect C1 8200) at a medical laboratory in Constantine. Included are: Blood glucose, creatinine, urea, albumin, bilirubin, total protein, Alanine Amino Transferase (ALAT), Aspartate Amino Transferase (ASAT), triglyceride and cholesterol.

2.4. Autopsy

Six animals from each batch are subjected to necropsy, involving macroscopic examination of the external surface of the body, all orifices, the cranial, thoracic and abdominal cavities and their contents. Liver and kidney samples are taken and preserved (10% formalin).

2.5. Histology

2.5.1. Technical

The methodology is explained and illustrated above.

2.5.2. Lesion readings

A reading grid (graded classification) is drawn up according to Jianmin Chen et al (2002), to facilitate the understanding of the lesions found and to be able to interpret them easily (Table XIV).

Regarding the morphological aspect of the liver and its components (hepatocytes, portal space, centrilobular vein) and the kidney (glomerulus, tubules), the cytoplasmic lesion classification is as follows:

-Preserved morphology=No lesions = 0

-From 1 to 3 (light, medium, heavy injury)

Table XIV: Lesion reading grid

Lesions	Score	Meaning
	0	Absence
	1	Legere
	2	Average
	3	Important

The classification of the lesion types: steatosis, fibrosis and inflammation of the liver and kidney, is graded from 0 to 3 (absent, slight, moderate, severe) respectively. The index of each lesion is calculated according to the formula of the same author, whose equation is adapted as follows: Index = (1x Number of rabbits+2xNumber+3xNumber)/total.

3. RESULTS

The parameters monitored for sub-chronic toxicity are the body weight of the rabbits in the different batches used, blood biochemistry and histological examination of the two filter organs: liver and kidneys.

3.1. Weight of rabbits

Weighing of this chapter (336) revealed that flaxseed supplementation did not block the growth of the rabbits, on the contrary, there was a highly significant increase (24%) between M0 and M3 (P=0.001). Thus, the similar increase (23%) in weight is significant (P=0.01) in the control lot. In contrast, there was no significant difference between the two batches at M3 (Table XV).

Table XV: Weight (g) of test rabbits: C2

	Witness	Seed	P

Mo	2530±300	2500±224	NS
M1	2760±270	2770±260	NS
M2	2930±280	2900±280	NS
M3	3110±280	3100±360	NS

NS: Not significant
S: Significant

3.2. Biochemical parameters

3.2.1. Monthly evolution

The observed means of various parameters (of each month) are shown in Figure 25. There was a significant decrease in glycemia of the seed lot compared to the control at M1 (P=0.042) and in creatinine at M2 (P=0.034), but a significant increase in triglycerides at M3 (P=0.023).

Monthly monitoring of the flax-supplemented rabbits shows a variation in biochemical parameters between Mo and M3 (Figure 26).

Indeed, the recorded rates of decrease in cholesterol (58%) and blood glucose (25%) showed a highly significant difference (P=0.03 and P=0.02).

The decrease in creatinine and albumin was 7.7% and 6.6% respectively with no significant difference (P>0.05).

In contrast, ASAT, urea, ALAT and total protein levels increased (without significant difference) by 29%, 26%, 22%, and 6.3% respectively.

3.2.2. General situation

The observed averages of various parameters are reported in Table XVI and illustrated in Figure 27. A decrease in the following parameters was observed: cholesterol (33%), creatinine (19%), urea (18%), blood glucose (13%), total protein (7%), AST (7%), albumin (4%) and bilirubin (3%), in the seed lot. In addition, an increase in mean triglycerides (21%) and ALT (17%) was recorded compared to the control lot. It is evident that statistically, no significant difference (P>0.05) is recorded for all the changes in blood biochemistry at general situation.

Table XVI: Average blood biochemical parameters

	Witness	Seed	P
Glyc (g/l)	1,31±0.28	1,14± 0.25	NS
Choles (g/l)	0,33±0,07	0,22±0,12	NS
Triglyc (g/l)	0,89±0,5	1,08±0,4	NS
ALT (U I/l)	29,78±14	34,92±16	NS
AST (UI/l)	28,67±29	26,54±17	NS
Biliru (mg/l)	0,5±0,4	0,57±0,4	NS

Prot (g/l)	60,89±3,5,	56,38±7,9	NS
Album (g/l)	42,56±10	40,69±14	NS
Uree (g/l)	0,51±0,64	0,42±0,37	NS
Crea (mg/l)	7,3±1,4	5,92±0,1	NS

NS: Not significant

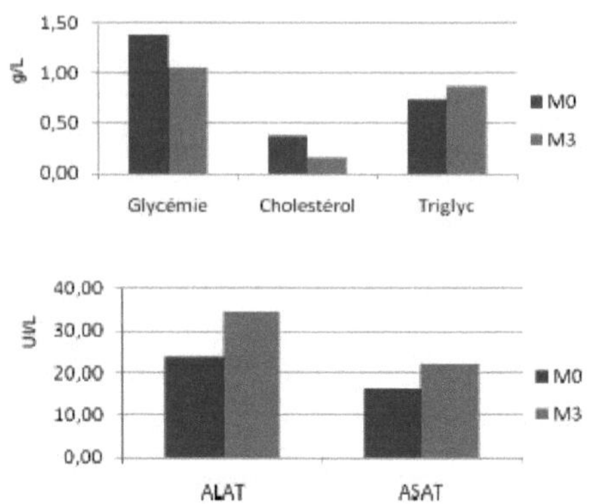

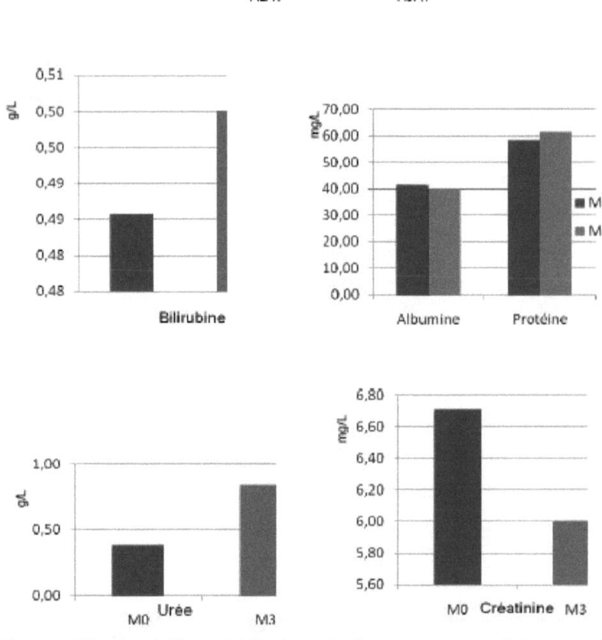

Figure 26: Evolution of biochemical parameters of the seed lot

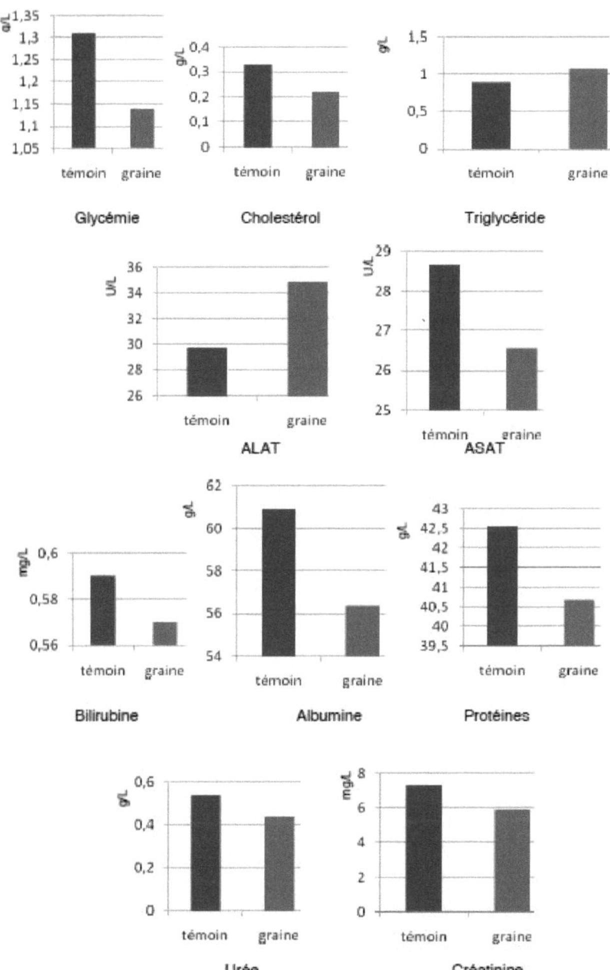

Figure 27: Average biochemical parameters of the two test batches C

3.3. Histology

At necropsy of the control lot, two rabbits showed respiratory lesions, but no lesions were observed in the seed lot.

Since some ingerates can alter any of the functions of the organs responsible for biotransformation and excretion (metabolism of a xenobiotic) and their constituents: (hepatocytes, portal spaces, centrolobular vein, glomeruli and tubules). Histological examination of liver and kidney sections revealed that the general appearance of the organs of the seed rabbits was similar to that of the control rabbits. Thus, it showed a preserved morphology (figure 28), while showing the absence of steatosis, inflammation and/or fibrosis.

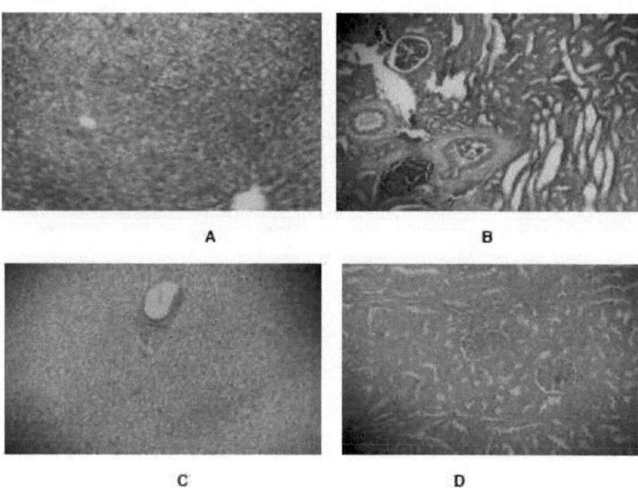

Figure 28: Microphotograph of the liver and kidney

A: Rabbit seed liver, **B**: Rabbit seed kidney, **C**: Rabbit control liver, **B**: Rabbit control kidney

No hepatic abnormalities were observed in the control lot. However, in the seed lot, a slight change in the hepatocyte was noted and a slight hepatic inflammation was observed in one rabbit (Table XVII).

Table XVII: Notification of liver lesions in the batches.

Type of lesion	Index	
	Sample lot	Seed lot
Overall morphology	0	0
Hepatocyte	0	0,83
Door space	0	0,16
Centro-lobular vein	0	0,70
Steatose	0	0
Fibrosis	0	0
Inflammation	0	0,16

The kidney lesion index was zero in rabbits from both batches for all elements considered: overall morphology, glomerulus tubule, fibrosis and inflammation (Table XVIII).

Table XVIII: Notification of renal lesions in batches

Type of lesion	Index	
	Sample lot	Seed lot
Overall morphology	0	0
Glomerulus	0	0
Tubule	0	0
Fibrosis	0	0
Inflammation	0	0

Finally, the hepato renal exploration of the study is coherent, since the biochemical blood data (ALT / ASAT / albumin / total protein and Urea / Creatinine) did not show any significant difference, for the liver and the kidney, confirming their histological integrity.

4. DISCUSSION

4.1. Clinical monitoring

In the present study, the choice of dose (1g/kg/D) is based on that used in the literature (Hermier et al, 2004).

Rabbits showed no signs of toxicity throughout the experimental period, only one rabbit had transient diarrhoea for three days during the adaptation period.

No abnormalities were found in the appetite and behaviour of the animals. No significant difference was observed in the body weight of the two batches (**_Seed_** and **_Control_**)

No significant difference was recorded in weight gain between the two batches, but the increase was significant between M_0 and M_3 in the seed batch. Our results are close to those reported by Djerrou, (2011); Halmi et al, (2013) and Maameri, (2014). Nevertheless, they are different from those reported by Ahmad et al, (2012) and Ognik et al (2012). This is probably related to the use of flaxseed and flaxseed oil extract by the latter two authors.

4.2. Biological monitoring

Analysis of blood parameters is relevant for risk assessment. Changes in the blood system have predictive value for human toxicity, when data are converted from animal studies (Tahraoui et al, 2010).

The results of the present study show that supplementation with flaxseed for 3 months had no significant effect on the majority of the parameters in the New Zealand rabbit. However, from the first month onwards, the seed caused a decrease in the majority of the parameters. These values are within the physiological norms as reported by Quinton (2003) and Archetti et al, (2008).

Average **blood glucose** and **cholesterol levels** were reduced in rabbits supplemented with flaxseed, which is in agreement with the results of Hermier et al, (2004) and Weill and Mairesse (2010).

Flax can be considered a "functional food", as it contains nutrients and other components such as polysaccharides, polyphenolics and beneficial essential fatty acids. Flax also contains 8% mucilage, which is a soluble fibre that can reduce the post-meal glycemic response and delay digestion and absorption of carbohydrates (Patterson, 2006). The hypoglycemic effect of *Linum usitatissimum* could thus be attributable to the presence of various polyphenols and polysaccharides in flax. Indeed, some flavonoids isolated from plants could have effects on glucose metabolism. They inhibit glucose transporters in the intestine, decrease the expression of genes that control neoglucogenesis, increase hepatic glucose storage and reduce glycogen (Waltner-loi et al, 2002; Shimizu et al, 2000; Li et al, 2004; Sarkhail et al, 2007). In addition, flavonoid extracts stimulate and regenerate pancreatic в cells (Esmaeili and Yazdanparas, 2004; Sharma et al, 2006; Shipra et al, 2009). Sarkhail et al (2007) report that polysaccharides and terpenes have a hypoglycemic effect.

In several organs, cellular lesions are followed by the release of a number of cytoplasmic enzymes into the bloodstream, a phenomenon that forms the basis for paraclinical diagnosis and biological monitoring (Sundberg et al, 1994; Dolai et al, 2012).

In our study, **liver function** was assessed by measuring plasma ALT and ASAT activity, albumin, and total protein concentration, which are indicators of hepatotoxicity (Manjeshwae et al, 2004; Tahraoui et al, 2010; Harizal et al, 2010; Atsamo et al, 2011).

Concerning transaminases, the results show an increase in **ALAT** (17%) and a decrease in **ASAT** (7%) in the seed lot. But these values remain without significant difference and within the physiological norms.

However, the level of these enzymes is significantly elevated, following a comparison of 500mg flaxseed/kg and 40ug/kg rastradiol, in laboratory rats (Ahmad et al, 2012).

Damage to the structural integrity of the liver results in an increase in liver-specific enzymes (ALT, ASAT) in serum, because they are cytoplasmic enzymes and sensitive to oxidative stress (Janbaz and Gilani, 1995; Venkateswaran et al, 1995; Das et al, 2010).

Flaxseed oil has antioxidant properties that probably result from the presence of lignans and some proteins (Bhatia et al, 2006, Barthlet et al, 2014). However, ingestion of flaxseed could have a hepatoprotective effect as reported by Faseehuddin Shakir and Madhusudhan (2007a). In rats with long-term exposure to azoximethane, Y-glutamyl transpeptidase, liver lipid profile and micronucleus formation were significantly reduced after receiving a flaxseed supplemented diet. This protection against oxidation may be related to the high amount of ligan secoisolariciresinal diglucoside in flax. The diet also caused a reduction in serum marker enzymes (Faseehuddin Shakir and Madhusudhan, 2007b).

Total protein and **albumin** were slightly decreased. These results are in agreement with those reported by Djerrou et al (2011).

Decreases in total plasma protein and albumin are proposed as indicators of altered protein synthesis (Kubena et al, 1993). A decrease in serum levels is usually the result of decreased protein synthesis by the liver or increased protein loss in the gut and kidney, another possible cause of albumin decrease may be due to malabsorption (Orhue et al, 2005).

Kidney function has been assessed by measuring plasma creatinine and urea levels (Davis and Berdt, 1994; Finco, 1997; Correges et al, 1998). An elevated blood urea level usually indicates glomerular damage. Thus, an elevated blood creatinine concentration is an indication of renal dysfunction (Franck, 1992). However, the small decreases obtained in **urea and creatinine**, could indicate a possible impact of flaxseed on protein metabolism. It should be noted that these variations also remained within the physiological limit and statistically without significant difference between the two batches.

The results obtained in supplemented rabbits are confirmed by the work of Ognik et al, (2012), Halmi et al (2013) using aqueous extract of *Opuntia ficus indica* using flaxseed oil and that of Abdou and Hassan, (2014) testing omega 3. In contrast Abdel Moneim et al (2012) and Maameri (2014) report a significant increase in urea and creatinine using flaxseed oil and mastic oil respectively.

Ahmad et al (2012) showed that aqueous methanol extract of flaxseed has no adverse effect on kidney function.

Given the additional support that animals are more sensitive to oral toxicity than humans (Tahraoui et al, 2010) and that the dose tested (1g/Kg body weight) was found to be non-toxic, the daily dosage could be more than 60 g in adults.

4.3. Tissue monitoring

New products are being added to the list of hepatotoxicity of phytotherapy every year. The spectrum of lesions and manifestations induced is very varied, reproducing a large part of the hepato-biliary diseases that are difficult to diagnose Larry (2005). Thus, the toxicity of certain plants, particularly renal toxicity, leads to acute tubular necrosis. Traditional remedies are incriminated in acute renal failure and may also aggravate pre-existing renal failure or cause complications (Lengani et al, 2009). Nevertheless, supplementation with antioxidant medicinal plants could be considered as a remedy for oxidative stress and renal injury (Rafieian-kopaei, 2013).

In our study, it is reasonable to emphasise that subchronic administration of the seed did not cause damage to the liver and kidneys. This is confirmed by the histological examination of the selected organs which shows normal structure, preserved morphology without the presence of dissociated tracts, no necrosis, no steatosis, nor severe hepatocyte alteration. The lesion index remained less than 1. Inflammation in a single rabbit with seed did not appear to be the cause. Obviously the risk is low compared to uninjured rabbits.

Thus normal glomerulus morphology and distal tubules are observed without any inflammatory or hemorrhagic lesions. This indicates that there are no significant disorders of the two organs responsible for biotransformation and excretion (metabolism of a xenobiotic) (Rose and Hodgson, 2004).

Abdel Moneim et al, (2011) in their study on lead acetate induced renal failure, reported that flaxseed oil administration effectively improved the histological structure of the lesional kidney, restored body weight loss and decreased serum creatinine and blood urea levels.

Ethanolic extract of *Linum usitatissimum* seeds provides renal protection by stimulating the renin-angiotensin system and causing inhibition of renal artery occlusion (Ghule et al, 2011, 2012).

Indeed, omega-3 fatty acids ameliorate lead acetate-induced hepatic and renal histological lesions (Abdou and Hassan, 2014). Paradoxically, in humans, a case of rhabdomyolysis is described in correlation with flaxseed consumption. The dosage was 6-10 mg per day once in the morning after breakfast for three months (Prasad et al. 2012).

It is concluded that the supplementation of flaxseed at a rate of 1g/kg in rabbits did not block growth, did not cause any change in the general behaviour of the animals. Thus, it did not reveal any significant difference in the blood biochemistry between the two batches and especially no hepato-nephrotic impairment. Some physiological disturbances were found. We noted an increase in ALT and triglycerides (17% and 21%) and a decrease in all other parameters, cholesterol at 33% and blood sugar at 13%. This is in favour of a positive impact of this seed on liver function, without any possible effect on protein metabolism and suggesting a hypoglycemic effect. This attests, on the one hand, to the anti-diabetic and anti-cholesterol effect of flax and, on the other hand, to the functional integrity of the liver and kidney; guaranteeing the non-toxicity of the seed and the harmlessness of its repeated and prolonged ingestion for three months.

However, further experimental trials are essential, with a larger sample size at different doses.

CHAPTER VIII: DETERMINATION OF ZOOTECHNICAL PERFORMANCE

In order to improve animal performance, while limiting the adverse effects of feeding on animal health, research into new feedstuffs is constantly being carried out. The use of linseed in rations allows for the improvement of animal products (Audureau, 2007). This feeding method takes into account consumer expectations and thus represents an opportunity for the agricultural sector (Rondia et al, 2003).

In order to determine the impact of flaxseed intake in the rabbits' ration on zootechnical performance (Test: C3); the monitoring of the weekly weight of the rabbits during the test: C2 allowed the calculation of the average daily gain, thus reducing the number of animals used in the different preclinical trials. Since both batches are sacrificed at the end of the experiment. The opportunity is taken to take the slaughter weight of the different compartments, which is used to estimate the slaughter yield and to know the effect of the seed on some performances in the rabbit.

1. **MATERIALS:** (Annex 11)

2. **METHODS**

The evaluation of the impact of ground flaxseed in the rabbits' ration on zootechnical performance (Test: C3) was organised as follows (figure 29):

1. The average daily gain is calculated from the individual records of the two batches of rabbits *(Seed, Control)* used in the previous test.

2. At slaughter, the weight of the different compartments is taken separately using an ordinary scale, especially for the carcass and fleece, and another precision scale for the offal (craur, liver and kidneys).

3. The slaughter yield is calculated in relation to the live weight and concerns the carcass, fleece and the various offal.

4. The data is analysed statistically.

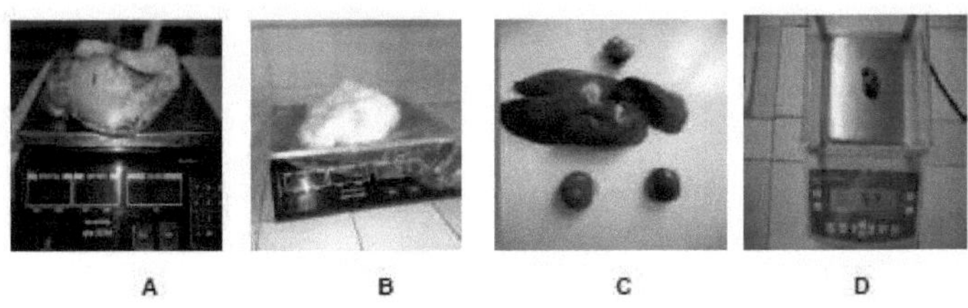

Figure 29: Assessment of slaughter yield
A: Carcass weighing, **B**: Fleece weighing, **C-D**: Examination and weighing of offal (gut, liver, kidneys)

3. **RESULTS**

In addition to average weight, average daily gain and slaughter yield (carcass, fleece, offal) are the criteria used for zootechnical performance after 13 weeks of flaxseed ingestion. The presence of respiratory lesions was reported at slaughter in two control animals.

3.1. Body weight

The weight of the rabbits is a classic parameter and is contained throughout the different trials conducted in the experimental stations. The different weekly weight averages obtained are presented in table XIX. It can be seen that there is no significant difference between the two batches. However, there is a highly significant increase in the average weight between s_1 and s_{13} (P=0.01 in the seed lot and P=0.004 in the control lot).

3.2. Average daily earnings

The evolution of the average daily gain is shown in figure 30. The GMQ in the control lot varies from 7g (s_1) to 3g (s_{13}), however, it varies from 16g (s_1) to 4.3g (s_{13}) in the seed lot. There is no difference in the variation of the average daily gain between the two batches.

Table XIX: Body weights (g) of both batches per week

	Witness	Seed	P
If	2600±270	2650±220	NS
S2	2650±300	2760±190	NS
S3	2620±260	2720±260	NS
S4	2760±270	2770±260	NS
S5	2820±190	2740±340	NS
S6	2880±220	2860±290	NS
S7	2850±240	2870±300	NS
S8	2930±280	2900±280	NS
S9	3000±260	3000±330	NS
S10	3050±280	3060±340	NS
S11	3030±280	3060±320	NS
S12	3090±290	3070±360	NS
S13	3110±280	3100±360	NS
P	0,004	0,01	

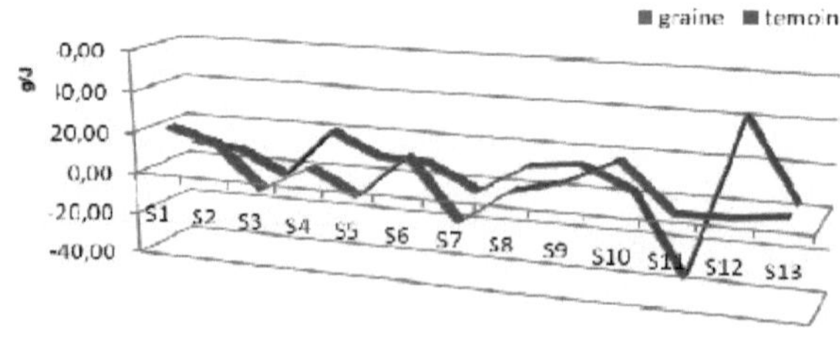

Figure 30: Evolution of the average daily gain of batches

3.3. Performance of the different compartments

The carcass weights of the two lots and their compartments are shown in Table XX.

g/j

98

The results show that there is a non-significant (P>0.05) decrease (1.2%) in the carcass of the seed lot compared to the control lot.

On the other hand, a slight decrease in fleece in the seed lot (1.04%) was noted. Concerning the weight of the different offal, a non-significant increase of 19% was observed in the seed lot.

Table XX: Average weight (g) of the different compartments

	Witness	Seed	P
Carcass	1732,5±183,8	1712,00±230,2	NS
Fleece	384,00±53,55	380,00±63,77	NS
Offal :	35,09±34,61	41,81±43,51	NS
Creur	7,891±1,271	9,636±2,613	NS
Liver	81,32±11,75	98,25±22,54	NS
Kidneys	16,056±1,562	17,543±3,393	NS

Figures 31 and 32 show the yield of the carcass and its different compartments. Values of 58% and 55% are obtained for the carcass yield of the control lot and the seed lot respectively. The offal yields of the control and seed lots were 3.67% and 4.02% respectively.

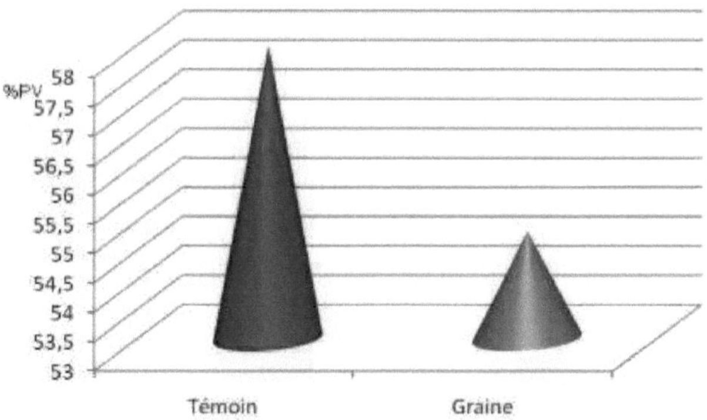

Figure 31: Assessment of carcass yield of batches

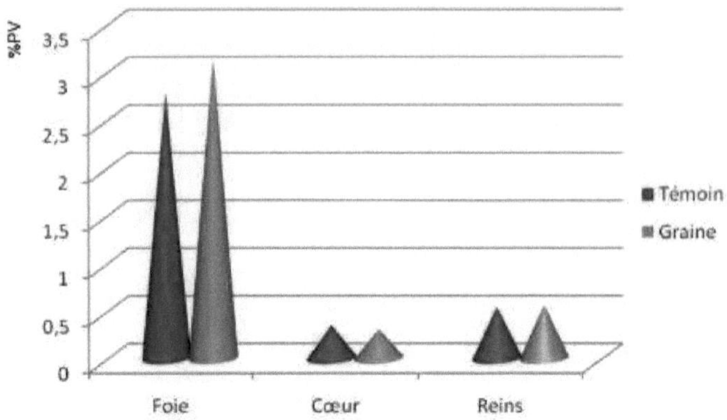

Figure 32: Assessment of offal yield

4. DISCUSSION

It should be noted that the gain in live weight over a short period of only 1-2 week(s) is almost twice as large as the gain in live weight in the same general situation (Lebas, 2010).

The supplementation with ground linseed did not influence live weight (at short interval and general situation), carcass weight or yields of anatomical elements to a significant extent at P<0.05.

This is in agreement with the work of Fomunyam et al (1985) who reported that breed and diet did not influence carcass quality. However, the kidneys of the maize-fed rabbits were significantly heavier than those of the cassava-fed animals, which is at variance with the data from the flaxseed supplemented rabbits.

The values obtained for carcass yields (55%-58%) are comparable to those (58%-60%) reported by Berchiche and Lebas (1994). However, they are higher than those reported by Fomunyam et al, (1985) with yields of 48% and 41%.

However, the ingestion of linseed did not significantly modify the average daily gain obtained (22g/d at s1 and 23g/d at s10). This is in agreement with the work of Ognik et al, (2012) who tested linseed oil on young hens. In contrast, Berchiche and Lebas (1994) reported QMGs of 33.7 to 60.1 g. This difference is probably due to the methionine supplementation of young growing rabbits, which is not the case with the present study where the rabbits are adults (24 weeks old).

Indeed, various studies have shown that the addition of fat to the end-of-fattening ration increases dry matter intake and GMQ. This increase in GMQ is even more pronounced when using extruded flaxseed compared to whole flaxseed, as the availability of nutrients is increased (Waylan et al, 2004; Maddock et al, 2006;

Labrune et al, 2008). The lack of significant difference between the two batches is probably due to the age of the rabbits (adult and not growing) and the presentation of the flaxseed (ground and not extruded).

Paradoxically, there does not seem to be any effect of w 3 fatty acid intake on the growth performance of rabbits or on body composition.

On the other hand, stronger or weaker correlations exist for the nutritional quality of rabbit meat (Benathmane et al, 2010).

Omega 3 fatty acids help to maintain a correct immune status of the animals due to their anti-inflammatory properties. A flaxseed-based diet rich in omega 3 helps to limit the development of pathologies, particularly respiratory ones, at the start of fattening, which is a "risk period" (Quinn et al, 2008). This can probably explain the presence of respiratory lesions found at autopsy in two control subjects and the absence of these lesions in the seed lot.

It is inferred that despite the low number of significant differences, this study was able to determine the impact of ground flaxseed supplementation on the weight of adult rabbits and on carcass performance and the different compartments. Indeed, an increase in weight between s_1 and s_{13} was highly significant (P=0.01) in the seed lot. The carcass yield of the seed lot (55%) was lower than that of the control lot (58%), but the offal yield (4.02%) was slightly higher.

However, other tests remain favourable, as to the nutritional quality of rabbit meat and its benefits on animal and human health, provided that extruded linseed and a large number of young rabbits are available.

GENERAL CONCLUSIONS

At the end of this study, we have tried to contribute to the enhancement of traditional medicine through the use of flax in order to achieve the preparation of accessible and effective remedies in the treatment of burns and hair loss.

Our work aimed at further developing the existing data on the virtues of flaxseed, through preclinical trials and para-clinical analyses to determine two main aspects of its therapeutic properties, namely the impact on the healing of burns and the effect on hair growth.

The results have proven several properties of linseed. Based on the principle of the preference of natural products over chemical industrial products, it is possible to replace the latter, especially those used for the healing of burns, by flaxseed oil which is equally effective and less expensive. Its biological properties, demonstrated *in vivo* (mainly due to the essential fatty acids and secondarily to the other components of the seed), thus confirm the traditional use of this plant in the treatment of burns and wounds.

As for the exploration of preparations based on this plant for the promotion of hair growth, the experimental data obtained on rabbits indicate that crude linseed oil has a positive effect on hair growth. The same promising effect is also observed after ingestion of the seed and is probably due to the flavonoids which act on hair growth by strengthening the walls of the small blood capillaries supplying the hair follicles. A significant increase in hair width is mainly obtained with the topical application of flaxseed oil for 04 weeks. A similar result is also noted after 13 weeks of daily ingestion of the seed. This growth in width then continues for a further 04 weeks after withdrawal of the supplementation.

The tested oral dose of the seed in the rabbit sub-chronic study is considered safe. In fact, the clinical and biological investigations, in addition to the autopsy of the rabbits, provide reassuring evidence of the safety of *L. usitatissimum*, whose prolonged consumption of the seed has been shown to have no harmful effect on the health of the animals, which further attests to its pharmacological value (without side effects).

In addition to the above-mentioned therapeutic (burning) and cosmetic (hair regrowth) effects, the addition of flax (rich in w-3 fatty acids) to the animals' diet significantly improves their performance during the growth period. However, the results show no impact on the live weight of adult rabbits (full growth), nor on their carcass weight, nor on the yields of the different compartments at slaughter.

In the future, two aspects will be developed:

-   The evaluation of the healing activity of polyunsaturated fatty acid chains extracted from the seed of *L. usitatissimum at* concentrations varying from those used in this work. The study will be further investigated by histological exploration of wound healing at regular intervals in combination with the determination of certain inflammatory reaction factors.

-    Phytochemical study of the oil to determine the composition of substances active in hair growth and formulate preparations with specific extracts. Further tests will be undertaken to determine the number and histological structure of hair follicles, the structure, texture and chemical composition of the hair, in order to compare the activity of linseed oil with that of extracts of other plants as well as other pharmaceutical and parapharmaceutical products.

-    Finally, other therapeutic virtues remain to be investigated in the hope of finding a place for this blue flower in modern pharmacology.

BIBLIOGRAPHIC REFERENCES

1. **Abdeldjalil MC, Benseguni A, Messai A, Boudebza A, Agabou A, Aimeur F and Benazouz H. 2012,** Healing effect of mastic oil on experimental burns in rats, 5eme journee internationale de medecine vétérinaire Constantine 15-16 mai

2. **Abdeldjalil MC, Benseguni A, Messai A, Agabou A F and Benazouz H. 2014,** Meddicinal use of *Pistacia lentiscus* fixed oil in Constantine province, northeast Algeria, Journal of Natural Product and Plant Resources **4** (1):48-51

3. **Abdel-Moneim AE, Dkhil MA and Al-Quraishy S. 2011,** The potential role of flaxseed oil on lead acetate-induced kidney injury in adult male albino rats, *African Journal of Biotechnology 10(8): 1436-1451*

4. **Abdelnour H, 2008,** Les plantes et les herbes medicinales, Noumidia edition, 187p

5. **Adhirajan N, Ravi KT, Shanmugasundaram N and Mary B. 2003,** In vivo and in vitro evaluation of hair growth potential of Hibiscus rosa-sinensis Linn, *Journal of Ethnopharmacology 88: 235-239*

6. **Adhirajan N, Ravi KT, Shanmugasundaram N and Mary B. 2003,** In vivo and in vitro evaluation of hair growth potential of Hibiscus rosa-sinensis Linn. *J. Ethnopharmacol* **88**: 235-239

7. **Aguerre H. 2004,** Les lambeaux cutanes axiaux chez le chat et le chien, etude bibliographique et clinique retrospective, *These de medecine veterinaire*, Universite Paul Sabatier, Toulouse, 152p

8. **Ahmad N, Rahman ZU, Akhtar N and Ali S. 2012,** Effects of aqueous methanolic extract of Flax seeds (Linum usitatissimum) on serum estradiol, progesterone, kidney and liver functions and some serum biochemical metabolites in immature female rats, *Pakistan Veterinary Journal, 32(2): 211215*

9. **Albert D. Atsamo, Telesphore. B. Nguelefack, Jacques. Y. Datte, Albert Kamany (2011),** Acute and subchronic oral toxicity assessment of the aqueous extract from the stem bark of *Erythrina senegalensis* DC (Fabaceae) in rodents, *Journal of Ethnopharmacology 134: 697-702*

10. **Alhaidari Z., Von Tscharner C. (1997),** Anatomy and physiology of the hair follicle in domestic carnivores, Pratique Medicale et Chirurgicale de l'Animal de Compagnie, 32, 181-194

11. **Ali M, Ansari SH.1997,** Hair care and herbal drugs, *Indian Journal of Natural Products 13, 3-5*

12. **Alkhalifah A, Alsantali A, Eddy Wang Bsc, Kevin J.M celwee and Jerry Shapiro. 2010,** Alopecia areata update. Part I. Clinical Picture, Histopathology, and Pathogenesis, *J. Am. Acad. Dermatol* **62**:177-88

13. **Allain D. 2007,** Fleece and Fibre Measurement in Angora Goats and Angora Rabbits. *http://www.macaulay.ac.uk/europeanfibre/effnnewlda.htm,* Accessed 14/01/12

14. **Andree MS.2011,** La cicatrisation indispensable a la survie ou une affection a la vie, *Le medecin du Quebec 46(10)*: 49-56

15. **Anonymous.2006,** Safety pharmacology studies of pharmaceuticals for human use. Guidance for Industry ICH theme S7A, *Health Canada, p20*

16. **Anonymous.2010,** Cultivated flax. *The free encyclopedia Wikipedia. Accessed on 13 /06/12*

17. **Anonymous.2011,** Histology of the skin and its appendages, *Semiological course CEDEF: College des Enseignants en Dermatologie de France. University of*

Lyon, : 1-31

18. **Anonyme.2012,** *L'ail : Contre la chute des cheveux et pour leur croissance,* Read more at Ladepeche de Kabylie, http://www.depechedekabylie.com/pause-digest/127071-contre-la-chute-des-cheveux-et-pour-leur-croissance.html#Pb0Leti13VuHTsGl.

19. **Aouina, F., Remili, I., 2013,** Preclinical evaluation of some biological effects of *Lepidium sativum L.* Master thesis. Department of animal biology. Universite de constantine1, Algerie. 70p

20. **Archetti I, Tittarelli C, Cerioli M, Brivio R, Grilli G and Lavazza A. 2008,** Serum chemistry and hematology values in commercial rabbits: Preliminary data from industrial farms in northern Italy, *9th World Rabbit Congress- June 10-13, Verrona-Italy: 1147-1151*

21. **Arvy L, More J. 1975,** Atlas d'histologie du lapin, *Ed. Maloine. Paris,13- 23p.308 pp*

22. **Asimus E. 2001,** Les plaies, *Cours de Pathologie Generale de Chirurgie, Ecole nationale veterinaire Toulouse*

23. **Atsamo AD., Telesphore. B. Nguelefack, Jacques. Y. Datte, Albert Kamany (2011),** Acute and subchronic oral toxicity assessment of the aqueous extract from the stem bark of *Erythrina senegalensis* DC (Fabaceae) in rodents, *Journal of Ethnopharmacology 134: 697-702.*

24. **Attipou K, Anoukoum T, Ayite A, Missohou K and James K.1998,** Treatment of wounds with honey. *Experience of the CHU of Lome, Medecine d'Afrique Noire 45(11): 658-660*

25. **Audureau D., 2007,** Evaluation technico-economique d'un apport de graine de lin extrudee dans la ration de vaches laitieres de quatre elevages des Pays de la Loire *These de Doctorat Veterinaire, Faculte de Medecine, Nantes, 140 p*

26. **Awe EO and Makinde JM. 2009,** The hair growth promoting effect of *Russelia equisetiformis, Journal of Natural Products 2:70-73*

27. **Bae J.S., K.H. Jang and H.K. Jin (2005),** Polysaccharides isolated from *Phellinus gilvus* enhances dermal wound healing in streptozotocin-induced diabetic rats, *Journal of Veterinary Science. 6: 161-164*

28. **Baie Hj S., K.A. Sheikh. 2000,** The wound healing properties of *Channa striatus-cetrimide* cream-wound contraction and glycosaminoglycan measurement, *Journal of Ethnopharmacology 73: 15-30*

29. **Bargues L, Carsin H.2003,** Comprendre et evaluer les brulures, in Goldestin P: les brulures. Cours d'Enseignement Superieur de Medecine. SFMU_LC 24/02/03 13:56, 47-62

30. **Barthet VJ, Klensporf-Pawlik D and Przybylski R. 2014,** Antioxidant activity of flaxseed meal components, *Canadian Journal of Plant Science 94: 593-602*

31. **Bauchart D, Anne de la Torre, Durand D,Gruffat D, Peyron A.2002,** L'apport de graine de lin ◁35▷ L'apport de graine de lin rich in linolenic acid favours the depot of CLA mainly in muscle triglycerides in steers, *9ᵉᵐᵉ journee des sciences du muscle et technologie de la viande. (15-16 OCTOBER.Clermont- Ferrand 73- 74*

32. **Bauchart D,Durand D,Mouty D,Dozias D,Ortigues-Marty I et Micol D.2001,** Effet d'un regime a base d'herbe sur la teneur et la composition en acides gras des lipides des muscles et du foie chez le bouvillon a l fatissement, *8ᵉᵐᵉ Journee,*

Rencontre, Recherche, Ruminants (5-6 Decembre, 2001). Communication 141.Paris

33. **Baudoux D.2003,** L'aromatherapie.se soigner par l'huile essentielle, *Edition Amyris*, 255p

34. **Baumann, L. and Spencer, J. 1999,** The effects of topical vitamin E on the cosmetic appearance of scars, Dermatologic Surgery. 25: 311-315

35. **Belfedle FZ.2009,** Huile de fruit de Pistacia lentiscus caracteristique physico-chimique et effet biologique (effet cicatrisant chez le rat), *Memoire presente pour obtenir le diplôme de magister en chimie organique.Option: phytochimie .Universite constantine,* 144p

36. **Beloued A.2009,** Les plantes medicinales en Algerie, *5eme edition 85p*

37. **Benatmane F, Kouba M, Fillaut M and Robin G. 2010,** Effect of flaxseed intake in the diet on the nutritional quality of rabbit meat, *13eme Journee des Sciences du Muscle et Technologie de la Viande*

38. **Benatmane F, Kouba M, Fillaut M, Robin G et Mourot J.2010,** Effet de l'apport de graines de lin dans le régime sur la qualite nutritionnelle de la viande de lapin, *I3^{(;me} journee des sciences du muscle et technologie de la viande,Revue des instituts de recherches et des centres techniques des filieres viandes et produits carnes*

39. **Benazzouz M.2001,** Evaluation des effets antibacteriens, antifongiques et de l'action cicatrisantes de *Lawsonia inermis L, These de doctorat d'etat en medecine vétérinaire, Option: chirurgie Universite Mentouri Constantine,* 120p

40. **Benlaksira B, Souheila S, Halmi Z,Djerrou K,Beroual K,Bachtarzi K ,Maamri Z and Hamdi Pacha Y.2013,** Cicatrizing effect of *Opuntia ficus-indica* aqueous extract and seeds powder in New Zealand rabbits, International Journal of Medicinal and Aromatic Plants 3(2):159-162

41. **Bensegni, A. 2007,** Les onguents traditionnels dans le traitement des plaies et des brulures. D. in veterinary sciences. Universite Mentouri Constantine, 2007, 107p

42. **Benseguni A, Belkhiri N, Boulebda G and Keck. 2007,** Evaluation of the healing activity of a traditional ointment from the Constantine region on excision wounds in rats, *Sciences & Technologie 26 :.83-87*

43. **Berchiche M, Lebas F.1994,** Supplementation en methionine d'un aliment a base de feverole : effets sur la croissance, le rendement a l'abattage, et la composition de la carcasse chez le lapin. *World Rabbit Science 2 (4) 135-140*

44. **Berglund DR. 2002,** Flax: New uses and demands. In Janick, J. and Whipkey, A, (Eds.). Trends in new crops and new uses, pp. 358-360, Alexandria: ASHS Press

45. **Bernard B. 2001,** Plantes medicinales du monde, 2ieme Edition,

46. **Bernard BA.2006,** The revealed life of the human hair follicle. *Medecine/Sciences 2 (22): 138-143*

47. **Bhatia AL, Manda K, Patni S and Sharma AL.2006,** Prophylactic Action of Linseed (Linum usitatissimum) Oil Against Cyclophosphamide-Induced Oxidative Stress in Mouse Brain, *Journal of medicinal food 9 (2): 261-264*

48. **Biswas T.K., L.N. Maity, B. Mukherjee. 2004,** Wound healing potential of *Pterocarpus santalinnus* Linn: a pharmacological evaluation. *The Internatinal Journal of Lower Extremity Wounds* 3: 143-150

49. **Bloedon LT and Szapary PO. 2004,** Flaxseed and cardiovascular risk, *Nutrition Review 62(1):18-27*

50. **Blumenthal MA, Goldberg J and Brinckmann EDS.2000,** Herbal Medicine: Expanded Commission E Monographs, American Botanical Council, Austin, TX, USA, pp 85

51. **Bong SU Kang, JA Seon Yoon, Dang-Young Kim, Jae-Hwang Jeong, EunYoung KIM, Sang Yoon Nam, Young Won Yun, Jong-Soo Kim, Beom Jun Lee.** 2011, Effects of Herbal Extracts on Hair Growth Promotion in Experimental Animal Mode. *Journal of Biomedical Research* **12**(2):113-120

52. **Boon HS, Olatunde F and Zick SM.2007,** Trends in complementary/alternative medicine use by breast cancer survivors: comparing survey data from 1998 and 2005, *BioMedCentral Womens Health*;7:4,1-7, http://www.biomedcentral.com/1472-6874/7/4

53. **Borel JP and Maquart F. 1998,** Mecanisme moleculaire de la cicatrisation des brulures, *Annales de -biologie, clinique,* **56** (1) :11-19

54. **Boukeloua A, Belkheri A, Djerrou Z, Behri L, Boulebda N and Hamdi-Pacha Y. 2012,** Acute toxicity of *Opucia ficus indica* and *Pistacia lentiscus* seed oils in mice, *African Journal of Traditional, Complementary and Alternative medicines 9(4):607-611*

55. **Boukeloua A.2009,** Caracterisation botanique et chimique et évaluation pharmacologique d'une préparation topique a base de l'huile de pistasia lentiscus.L (*ANACARDIACEAE), Memoire en vue de l'obtention du diplôme de magister en biologie, specialite: biotechnologie végétale. Universite Mentouri Constantine1*, 108p

56. **Boulebda N,Belkheri A,Belfadel FZ,Benseguni A and Bahri L. 2009,** Dermal wound healing effect of *Pistacia lentiscus* fruit's fatty oil, *Pharmacognosy Research 1(2): 66-71*

57. **Bourges-Abella N. (2008),** La peau des mammiferes, *Cours dhistologie S5 de l'Ecole Nationale Veterinaire de Toulouse, 53p*

58. **Bourin M.1991,** Pharmacologie generale, 4eme edition Paris ; p 304

59. **Bourre JM. 2004,** Psychiatry and dietary omega-3 fatty acids, Medicine and Nutrition **40**: 171-182

60. **Boutaleb, H., 2014,** Evaluation of the healing effects of *Teucrium polium* on excision wounds in rats. Memoire de magistere. Institut des Sciences Veterinaires. Universite de Constantine 1. Algerie 140p

61. **Boutonnat J. 2008,** La peau, *Cours d'histologie, Faculte de medecine de Grenoble.* Available on Linkurlhttp://umvf.biomedicale.unparis5.fr/wiki/docvideos/Grenoble_0708/BOU TONNAT_Jean/BOUTONNAT_Jean_P01/BOUTONNAT_Jean_P01.p

62. **Branswyck J. 2009,** Prescription tool for modern dressings. 72 P, *www.urml-reunion.net/fmc/pansementsmodernes_branswyck.pdf. Accessed on 10/08/2010*

63. **Breathnach A and Bannister LH. 1995,** Integumental system, skin and breasts,*In* Gray's anatomy *(Williams, P.L, Ed) pp. 376-412, Churchill- Livingstone, New-York.*

64. **Brenner J.2003,** Essential Fatty Acids and the Skin, *Bioriginal Food & Science Corp 1-5*

65. **Broeck WV, Mortier P and Simoens P.2001,** Scanning electron microscopic study of different hair types in various breeds if rabbits, *Folia Morphol **60**(1):33- 40*

66. **Bruant-Rodier C.2005,** Cicatrisation et traitement des pertes de substances cutanees etendues, *U. L.P.- Faculte de Medecine Strasbourg - DCEM1 2004/ 2005 - Module 12B - Appareil Locomoteur, 18p*

67. **Bruneton J. 1987,** Element de photochimie et pharmacognosie .technique et documentation, *Edition Lavoisier, 585p*

68. **Bruneton J. 1993,** Pharmacognosy, photochemistry, medicinal plants, 3eme edition. Lavoisier, Paris, 915p

69. **Brunschig P, Kernen P et Weill P.1997,** Effet de l'apport d'un concentrate enrichi en acides gras polyinsatures sur les performances de vaches laitieres a l'ensilage de maïs, *Rencontre, Recherche, Ruminants, 4 : 361*

70. **Buhl AE.1989,** Minoxidil's action in hair follicles, *J Invest Dermatol* **92**:315320

71. **Canadian EGG Marketing Agency.2007,** Omega-3 enriched eggs. Canadian Egg Marketing Agency, Accessed: April 28,   2008, http://www.eggs.ca/pdf/omega-3_e.pdf, Sensory evaluation of flaxseed of different varieties. In Proceedings of the 56th Flax Institute of the United States, pp. 201-203. Fargo North Dakota: Flax Institute of United States

72. **Shah K.F., C.A. Eze, C.E. Emuelosi and C.O. Esimone 2006,** Antibacterial and wound healing properties of methanolic extracts of some Nigerian medicinal plants, *Journal of Ethnopharmacology* 104: 164-167

73. **Chari Z.1999,** Effet cicatrisants d'*Inula viscosa* sur les brulures experimentales chez le lapin, Diplome de magister Universite Mentouri .Constantine, 97p

74. **Charroufa Z et Guillaumeb D. 2007,** Huile d'argan une production devenue adulte. Article de synthèse, *Les technologies de laboratoire N°6.pp 6.*

75. **Chen J, Stavro PM, Thompson LU. 2002,** Dietary flaxseed inhibits human breast cancer growth and metastasis and downregulates expression of insulinlike growth factor and epidermal growth factor receptor, *Nutrition and Cancer* **43**(2):187-192

76. **Chesneau G, Quemener B, Weill P. 2004,** Qualite nutritionnelle des lipides de viande, ecart lies a l'espece, ecarts lies a L'alimentation, quelques observations, *io$^{(;me}$ Journee des sciences du muscle et technologie de la viande, Rennes, 59-60*

77. **Chilliard Y,Ferlay A,Mansbridge RM and Doreau M.2000,** Ruminant Milk fat plasticity nutritional control of saturated, polyunsaturated Trans and conjugated fatty acids, *Annales de Zootechnie* **49**: 181-205

78. **Choi S.W., B.W. Son, Y.S. Son, Y.I. Park, S.K. Lee, M.H. Chung (2001),** The wound healing effect of a glycoprotein fraction isolated from *Aloe vera*. British *Journal of Dermatology 145: 535-545*

79. **Choiniere M.2000,** Le point sur le traitement de la douleur chez les patients brules, *Brulures, 1(3) :128-135*

80. **Chong CM,Nickoloff BJ,Elias PM,Goldsmith LA,Macher E,Maderson PA,Sundberg JP,Tagami H,Plonka PM,Thestrup-Pederson K,Bernard BA,Schroder JM,Dotto P,Chang CM,Williams ML,Feingold KR,King LE, Kligman AM, Rees JL and Christophers E.2002,** What is the 'true' function of skin? Exp.Dermatol. 11: 159-187

81. **Chuong CM, Hou L, Chen PJ, WU P, Patel N and Chen Y. 2001,** Dinosaur's feather and chicken's tooth? Tissue engineering of the integument, European Journal of Dermatology 11,286-292

82. **Clere N. 2010,** Hair loss, how to prevent or slow it down? *Actualite Pharmaceutique 500: 32-34*

83. **Clinquart A,Micol D,Brundseaux C, Dufrasne I and Istasse L. 1995,** Utilisation des matieres fattes chez les bovins a l'engraissement, *INRA Production Animale, 8(1), 29-42*

84. **Collin M,Raguenes N, Le Berre G,Charrier S,Pringent AY et Perrin G. 2005,** Influence d'un enrichissement de l'aliment en acides gras omega 3 provenant de graines de lin extrudees (Tradi-Lin®) sur les lipides et les caracteristiques hedoniques de la viande de Lapin, *ii^{emes} Journees de la Recherche Cunicole, 29-30 novembre, Paris*

85. **Commo S and Bernard BA.1997,** The distribution of alpha 2 beta 1, alpha 3 beta 1 and alpha 6 beta 4 integrins identifies distinct subpopulations of basal keratinocytes in the outer root sheath of the human anagen hair follicle, *Cell mol life Sci 5 :466-71*

86. **Corbu A.2008,** Synthese de Produits Naturels a Activite Biologique Importante Iridal, Acide Galbanique, Marneral et analogues, *This paper was presented to obtain the degree of Doctor of the Ecole POLYTECHNIQUE speciality: Chimie Organique. Paris,* 461p

87. **Correges JP, Becha J, Abood E, Andre L, Lamarka R. 1998,** Renal artery stenosis and chronic renal failure in NIDDM, *Archives of Heart and Vascular Diseases 91: 1077-1088*

88. **Coskuner Y, Karababa E. 2007,** Some physical properties of flaxseed (*Linum usitatissimum* L.), *Journal of Food Engineering. 78, 1067-1073*

89. **Costagliola M. 2011,** General principles of reconstructive surgery for burn injuries. *Annals of Aesthetic Plastic Surgery 56(5):354- 357*

90. **Cotsarelis G, Millar, SE. 2001,**Towards a molecular understanding of hair loss and its treatment, *Trends in Molecular Medicine 7:293-301*

91. **Coulibaly SL.2008,** Contribution a revaluation de la qualité des medicaments traditionnels ameliores. *These d'application en Pharmacie, Faculte de Medecine de Pharmacie et d'Odonto-stomatologie, Universite de Bamako,* 90p

92. **Courtin-Donas S. 2009,** Peau et pelage du chien, *Actualites pharmaceutiques 483 :46-48*

93. **Cronin RH and Henrich WL. 2005,** Toxic nephropathies, in HILLAL G, ALBERT C, VALLEE M 2005, Mecanisme impliques dans la nephrotoxicite, *Annales de Biologie Clinique, Quebec 42 (3):29*

94. **Dadoune JP,Hadjiisky P,Siffroi JP, Vendrely F. 2007,** Histologie, deuxièmeieme edition, Flammarion, 450p

95. **Dallezotte A. 2000,** Proprietes specifiques de la viande de Lapin, *Jornadas internacionales de cunicultura, Vila Real (Portugal), 24-25 November*

96. **Das SK, Mukherjee S, Gupta G, Rao DN and Vasudevan DM.2010,** Protective effect of resveratrol and Vitamin E against ethanol -induced oxidative damage in mice, *Indian Journal Biochemist Biophysics: 47(1): 32-37*

97. **Daun J, Barthet V, Chornick T and Duguid S.2003,** Structure, composition, and variety development of flaxseed, *In: Thompson, L., Cunanne, S. edition. Flaxseed in Human Nutrition. 2nd edition Champaign, Illinois. pp.1-40*

98. **Davis ME and Berdt WD. 1994,** Renal methods for toxicology, *In Hayes, A.W.*

(eds) Principles and methods of toxicology, 3rd Ed. New York Raven, pp. 871894

99. **Deloche C, de Lacharriere O, Mischiali C, Piraccini BM, Vincenzi C, Bastien P, Tardy I, Bernard BA and Tosti A.2004,** Histological features of peripilar signs associated with androgenetic alopecia. *Archives of Dermatological Research* **295** : *422-8.*

100. **Delverdier M,Bret L,Raymond I et Magnol JP.1993,** La réaction inflammatoire : secondaire .dynamique et signification biologique, *Prat Med Chir Anim Comp* **28**:*589-603*

101. **Deodhar AK, Rana RE.1997,** Surgical physiology of wound healing: *A review,* Journal of Postgraduate. Medicine, 43(2): 210-212

102. **Derek J. Ruthig and Kelly A. Meckling-Gill, 1999,** Both (n-3) and (n-6) Fatty Acids Stimulate WoundHealing in the Rat Intestinal Epithelial Cell Line, IEC-6. Journal of Nutrition, 129, 1791-1798

103. **Descamps H, Baze Delecroix C and Jauffret E. 2001,** Reeducation de l'enfant brule. Encyclopedie de la Medico- Chirugicale Kinesitherapie - Medecine physique-Readaptation, *Editions Scientifiques et Medicales Elsevier SAS, Paris),* D(10), 26-275 P

104. **Dhennin C. 2002,** Local treatment of burns, *Pathology Biology **50**(2): 109-117*

105. **Diederichsen A and Richards K.2003,** Cultivated flax and the genus Linnum L.: taxonomy and gerplasm conservation, *In Muir, A. D. and Westcott, N. D. (Eds). Flax, The genus Linum, pp. 22-54. London: Taylor & Francis*

106. **Dif RH,Lalonde CL and Bret L. 2010,** Restoration and maintenance of hemodynamic stability, *In burn trauma, trauma management IV. Edition: Blaisdell and Turnkey. New York, 24- 39*

107. **Diouri M,Chafiki N,Mradmi W,Bahechar N and Boukind EH.2003,** La brulure : une plaie pas comme les autres : Elements epidemiologiques, physiopathologiques, diagnostiques, Esperance medicale **10**(95):301-306

108. **Djago A.Y., Kpodekon M., Lebas F., 2010,** Le guide pratique de l'éleveur de lapins sous les tropiques, 2eme edition. *Cecuri ed, Abomey-Calavi (Benin) 116 pages*

109. **Djenane R.1997,** Les brulures, Revue de la formation continue des professionnels de la sante **6**: 5-10

110. **Djerrou Z, Maamari Z, Hamdi-Pacha Y,Serakta M, Riachi F, Djaalab H and Boukeloua A. 2010,** Effect of virgin fatty oil of *Pistacia lentiscus* on experimantal burn wound's healing in rabbits, African Journal of Traditional, Complementary and Alternative 7(3): 258-263

111. **Djerrou Z.2011,** Effects of some natural molecules in medicine: healing and innocuousness activity of the vegetable oil of *Pistacia lentiscus L.* These de Doctorat en Sciences. Department of Veterinary Sciences. Universite Mentouri de Constantine, Algerie. 157p

112. **Djerrou Z, Maamari Z, Hamdi-Pacha Y, Belkhiri B, Djaalab H, Riachi F, Seraktaa A, Boukeloua A and Maameri Z. 2011,** Evaluation of *pistacia lentiscus* fatty oil effects on glycemic index, Liver functions and kidney functions of new zealand rabbits, African Journal of Traditional, Complementary and Alternative 8(S):214-219

113. **Djerrou Z, Djaalab H, Riachi F, Serakta A, Chettoum Z,Maameri, Boutobza**

Z and Hamdi-Pacha Y,2013a, Irritantcy potential and sub-acute dermal toxicity study of *pistacia lentiscus* fatty oil as a topical traditional remedy, African Journal of Traditional, Complementary and Alternative 10(3) 480-489

114. **Djerrou Z, Bensari C, Bachtarzi K, Djaalab H, Riachi F, Maameri Y and Hamdi-Pacha Y.2013b,** Safety and efficacy of *Pistacia lentiscus* L. fruit's fatty oil for the treatment of dermal burns: A synthesis report, International Journal of Medicinal and Aromatic Plants 3(4): 464-469

115. **Djerrou Z. 2014,** Efficacy of honey bee and *Fagopyrum esculentum* Moench ointment in the treatment of sub chronic wound in rabbits: a case control study, American Journal of Animal and Veterinary Sciences **9** (1): 14-18

116. **Dos Tavares Pereira, DS., Maria Helena Madruga Lima-Ribeiro, Ralph Santos-Oliveira,Carmelita de Lima Bezerra Cavalcanti, Nicodemos Teles de Pontes-Filho,5 Luana Cassandra Breitenbach Barroso Coelho, AnaMaria dos Anjos Carneiro-Le~ao, Maria Tereza dos Santos Correia,** 2012, Development of AnimalModel for Studying Deep Second-Degree Thermal Burns Journal of Biomedicine and Biotechnology Volume 2012, Article ID 460841, 1-7 doi:10.1155/460841. Accessed 06/08/14

117. **Dscamps V, Bonnetblanc JM, Crickx B and Roujeau JC. 2002,** Examen national classant; maladies et grands syndromes: troubles des phaneres, Ann Dermatol Venereol **129**:2s194-2s198

118. **Dumas C,Kalonji E, Thomann C and Gnanou JC.2003,** Acides gras de la famille omega 3 et systeme Cardiovasculaire: interets nutritionnels et allegations, *A.F.S.A.A; editeur, Nancy, 124 pages*

119. **Duquennoy MV. 2009,** Normal and pathological wound healing: Notions on dressings. College hospitalier et universitaire de chirurgie pediatrique Paris, *Cours de diplome d'etudes specialises complementaires,76 DPR*

120. **Durand D, Gruffat Mouty D, Hocquette JF, Micol D, Dubroeucq H, Jailler S, Jadhao SB, Scislowski V and Bauchart D.2001,** Influence de la supplementation de la ration en huiles végétales riches en acides gras polyinsatures sur la lipoperoxydation plasmatique et musculaire chez le bouvillon en finition, *Journees, Rencontre, Recherche, Ruminants.175-178*

121. **Dweck, AC. 2002,** Herbal medicine for the skin - their chemistry and effects on skin and mucous membranes,Personal Care Magazine; 3:19-21

122. **Dyerberg J.1986,** Linolenate-derived polyunsaturated fatty acids and prevention of atherosclerosis. *Nutrition Reviews* **44**(4):125-134

123. **Ebling FJG.1987,**The biology of hair, *Dermatologic Clinics* **5**:*467-481*

124. **Echinard C and Latarjet J. 1993,** Les brulures, *ED. Masson, pp 23-35, 75-84*

125. **Eichele K.2010,** Phytotherapy-An introduction, *The Journal of the European Medical Writers Association (JEMWA) 19 (1): 67*

126. **Enoch, S., John Leaper. D. 2005,** Basic science of wound healing. Surgrery 23, (2):37-42

127. **Esmaeili MA, Yazdanparas R.2004,** Hypoglycemic effect of *Teucrium polium*: 265 studies with rat pancreatic islets. *Journal of Ethnopharmacology* **95**:*27- 266*

128. **Eugene M, Martin C, Mialon MM, Krauss D, Renand G and Doreau M. 2009,** Reduction of methane emissions in early fattening bulls fed with concentrate-rich rations supplemented with linseed. *1&! me Journee Rencontre Recherche*

Ruminants, Clermont- Ferrand, 2-3 December

129. **Fabre-Record F. 1982,** *Plantes et cicatrisation, These d'exercice. Pharmacie. Universite Montpellier I. UFR des sciences pharmaceutiques et biologiques. 103p*

130. **Faestvedt E and Stashak TS.2008,** Topical wound treatments and wound care products, *In: STASHAK, T.S THEORET C.L equine wound management Wiley Blackwell (Ed): 137- 159*

131. **Faseehuddin Shakir and Basavaraj M.2007a,** Effects of flaxseed (Linum Usitatissimum) chutney on gamma-glutamyl transpeptidase and micronuclei profile in azoxymethane treated rats, *Clinical of Biochemistry* Indian Journal *22: 129-131*

132. **Faseehuddin Shakir and Madhusudhan B.2007b,** Hypocholesterolemic and hepatoprotective effects of flaxseed chutney: evidence from animal studies, *Indian Journal of Clinical Biochemistry 22 (1): 117-121*

133. **Fayolle P. 1992,** Plaies par brulures: particularites physiopathologiques et therapeutiques, Le point vétérinaire: Chirurgie plastique et reconstructrice cutanee) **24**:467-474

134. FELASA 2007: Working Group on Ethical Evaluation of Animal Experiments, Principles and Practice in Ethical Review of Animal Experiments across Europe: A report of the Federation of European Laboratory Animal Science Associations (FELASA). *Laboratory Animals*;41:143-160

135. **Ferraq MY. 2007,** Developpement d'un modle de cicatrisation epidermique apres une desepidermisation laser, *These pour obtenir le grade de docteur Discipline: ingenierie medicale et biologique universite Toulouse IIII- PAUL SABATIER Toulouse U.F.R medicine, page 28, 32*

136. **Finco DR. 1997,** Kidney function, *In: Kanetto, J.J. Harvey, J.W., Bruce. M.L., editors. Clinical Biochemistry of domestic animal. 5th ed. San Diego, CA: Academic Press :462 - 478*

137. **Fomunyam RT, Adegbola AA and Oke OL.1985,** Cassava diet for rabbits, *Proceedings of the Second Triennial Symposium of the International Society for Tropical Root Crops - Arr/que Branch, 14-19 August 1983, Doliala, Cameroon*

138. **Fournier N and Mordon S.2005,** Nonablative remodeling with a 1,540 nm erbium: glass laser, *Dermatologic Surgery 31:1227-35*

139. **Foweler D.1993,** Principal of wound healing in harary. J:surgical complication and wound healing, *In the small animal practice philadephia, saunders W.B (13)*

140. **Frank C. Lu.1992,** Toxicology, general data, evaluation procedures, target organs, risk assessment, *Ed: Masson, 256p*

141. **Freeman TP .1995,** Structure of flaxseed. In: Cunnane S, Thompson LU *(Eds) Flaxseed in human nutrition. AOCS Press, Champaign Illinois, pp. 11-21*

142. **Frekha M. 1988,** La cicatrisation des plaies, *These d'exercice. Pharmacie. Universite Montpellierl.UFR des sciences pharmaceutiques et biologiques, 102p*

143. **Fuchs E, Merrill BJ, Jamora C, Dasgupta R. 2001,** At the roots of a neverending cycle. Devlopmental Cell 1(1): 13-25,

144. **Gagnon V. 2005,** Etude des interactions entre les nerfs sensoriels et les follicules pileux dans un modele in vitro de peau reconstruite par genie tissulaire, Memoire de maitrise en biologie cellulaire et moleculaire. Faculte de medecine universite Laval Quebec, 215p

145. **Galcera FC.2002,** Hair lotion useful for treatment of hair loss and stimulation

hair growth.United states patent ,US 6,447,762 B1

146. **Ganorkar PM and Jain RK. 2013,** Flaxseed - a nutritional punch: *International Food Research Journal 20(2): 519-525*

147. **Gentz EJ, Harreustien LA and Carpenter JW. 1995** Dealin gwith gastrointestinal, genitourinary and musculoskeletal problems in rabbits, symposium on rabbit medicine, *Medicine Veterinary 90(4): 365- 372*

148. **Geras, A. J. 1990.** Dermatology. A Medical Artist's Interpretation. Switzerland, Sandoz Medical Publications, 107p

149. **Ghileb GM. 1987,** Les plantes dans la medecine traditionnelle maghrebine.*Memoire de diplome d'etude en phytotherapie Tunis, 111p*

150. **Ghule AE, Jadhav SS and Bodhankar SL.2011,** Renoprotective effect of Linum usitatissimum seeds through haemodynamic changes and conservation of antioxidant enzymes in renal ischaemia-reperfusion injury in rat, *Arab Journal of Urology 9:215-221*

151. **Ghule AE, Jadhav SS and Bodhankar SL.2012,** Effect of Ethanolic Extract of Seeds ofLinum usitatissimum (Linn.) on Hemodynamic Changes and Left Ventricular Function in Renal Artery Occluded Renovascular Hypertension in Rats, *Pharmacologia 3 (8): 283-290*

152. **Gillmour J, Harrison C, Asadi L, Cohen MH and Vohra S.2011,** Natural health product-drug interactions: evolvingresponsibilitiesto take complementary and alternative medicine into account *Pediatrics 128 (4): S155- 60*

153. **Goodman LS and Gilman A.1996,** The pharmacological Basis of Therapeutics *Eds. New York, McGraw Hills; 1611*

154. **Grimbert A. 2009,** Cicatrisation des plaies aigues et chroniques, *Journee de la sante France. 36 DPR*

155. **Grosjean N. 2007,** Guide de traitement par les plantes medicinales et phytocosmetologie, *Edition heures de France vol 1, Paris*

156. **Guedje NM, Tadjouteu F, Dongmo RF, Jiofack RBT, Tsabang N, Fokunang CN, Fotso S.2012,** African Traditional Medicine (ATM) and Phytomedicines: Challenges and Development Strategies, Health Sciences and Disease 12 (3): 1-25

157. **Guenette L, Gilles P and Dioenne JY.2009,** Produits de sante naturels et medicaments, Un cocktail souvent benefique, *Revue Vitalite-Quebec,CANADA N°. 126*

158. **Guihard J. 2011,** Interets d'une supplementation en acides gras, omega-3 sur la production et la sante des vaches laitieresThese *d'exercice, Medecine veterinaire, Ecole Nationale Veterinaire de Toulouse85 p*

159. **Guilbaud J, Carsin H and Le Gulluche Y.1993,** Brulures, *Editions techniques. Encycl. Med. Chir. Therapeutique (Paris France). 25-712-A.pp1-12*

160. **Guillevic M, Mairesse G, Weill P, Guibert JM, Chesneau G et Valorex. 2010,** Un apport en graines de lin extrudees chez le poulet et la dinde Participe a l'amelioration de la qualite nutritionnelle de la Viande, *13³ᵐˢ Journee des sciences du muscle et technologie de la viande. Clermont-Ferrand. Review of the research institutes and technical centres of the meat and meat products sectors*

161. **Habbu PV, Joshi H and Patil BS.2007,** Potential wound healers from plant origin, *Pharmacognosy Reviews 1 (2): 271-281*

162.   **Habbu PV, Joshi H, Patil BS. (2007),** Potential wound healers from plant origin,*Phamacognosy Reviews 1(2): 271-281*

163.   **Hadshiew IM, Kerstin F, Petra C, Arck W and Ralf P.2004,** Burden of hair loss: Stress and the underestimated psychosocial: Impact of telogen effluvium and androgenetic alopecia, *J Invest Dermatol **123**:455-457*

164.   **Halligudi N.*2012,*** Pharmacological properties of flax seed: Review Hygeia: journal for drugs and medicines *vol **4** (2): 70-77*

165.   **Halmi S, Almi S, Benlakssira B, Bechtarzi Z,Beroual K, Serakta A, Riachi F, Djaalab H, Maameri Z, Djerrou Z, Hamdi Pacha Y.2013,** Pharmaco- toxicological study of *Opuntia ficus indica* L. aqueous extract in experimental animals, *J. Med. Arom. Plants ***3**(3): 375-381

166.   **Halmi S, Benlakssira B, Bechtarzi Z, Djerrou H, Djeaalab H, Riachi F and Hamdi Pacha. 2012,** Antihyperglycemic activity of prickly pear (*Opuntia ficus- indica*) aqueous extract. International Journal of Medicinal and Aromatic **Plants2**(3): 540-543

167.   **Hamdi Pacha Y, Benazzouz M, Belkhiri A, Chari Z, Serakta A. 1998 a,** Healing effect of lawsonia inermis, case of 3rd degree burns, Revue, Medecine pharmaceutique d'Afrique 11-12

168.   **Hamdi Pacha Y, Benazzouz M, Serakta A, Chari Z, Bensegueni L, Belkhiri A.1998 b,** Biological and pharmacological effect of some natural molecules: healing effect of *Inula viscosa* L, *Lawsonia inermis*, 15eme *congres veterinaire maghrebin, Cedre d'atlas genevrier, pin d'Alep a hammet (Tunisie) le 5 et 6 Mai*

169.   **Hamdi Pacha Y, Belkhiri A, Benazzouz M, Benhamza L, Bensegueni L. 2002,** Evaluation of the healing activity following experimental burns of some Algerian plants, *Revue Med. Pharm. Afri'*, **16:** 1-7.

170.   **Hamdi-Pacha Y, Benazzouz M, Kerrour M. 1995,** Nectar of *kniphofia uvularia moench*: effect on the healing process of burn wounds 3eme degree, Maghreb veterinaire

171.   **Hans koth W.2007,** 1000 plantes aromatiques et medicinales, edition terre for the french version, 300p

172.   **Harada N, Okajima K, Arai M, Kurihara H, Nakagata N. 2007,** Administration of capsaicin and isoflavone promotes hair growth by increasing insulin-like growth factor-I production in mice and in humans with alopecia, *Growth Horm. IGF Res. **17**:408-415*

173.   **Harada N and Okajima K. 2007,** Effect of topical application of capsaicin and its related compounds on dermal insulin-like growth factor-I levels in mice and on facial skin elasticity in humans, *Growth Horm. IGF Res. **17**:171-176*

174.   **Harada N, Okajima K, Narimatsu N, Hiroki K and Nakagata N. 2008,** Effect of topical application of raspberry ketone on dermal production of insulin-like growth factor-in mice and on hair growth and skin elasticity in humans, *Growth Hormone & IGF Research **18**:335-344*

175.   **Hardy MH.1992,** The secret life of the hair follicle, Trends Genet. 8, 55-61

176.   **Harizal SN, Mansor SM, Hasnan J, Tharakan JKJ and Abdullah J.2010,** Acut toxicity study of the standardized methanolic extract of *Mitragyna speciosa* Korthin Rodent, *Journal of ethnopharmacology **13**: 404-409*

177.   **Harrison CA, Gossiel F, Bullock AJ, Sun T, Blumsohn A and Mac neil**

S.2006, Investigation of keratinocyte regulation of collagen I synthesis by dermal fibroblasts in a simple in vitro model,Brit. *J. Dermatol* **154**: 401-410

178.   **Hattori M and Ogawa H.1983,** Biochemical analysis of hair growth from the aspects of aging and enzyme activities. *J Dermatol* **10**:45-54

179.   **He D.2006,** Bilan des connaissances actuelles sur la cicatrisation des plaies cutanees chez le chien et le chat, Memoire de docteur veterinaire *l'Universite Paul-Sabatier de Toulouse 234p*

180.   **Heba MA, Mohamed AH.2014,** Protective Role of Omega-3 Polyunsaturated Fatty Acid against Lead Acetate-Induced Toxicity in Liver and Kidney of Female Rats, *BioMedicinale Research International Article ID 435857: 1-11*

181.   **Heli Jroy RD, Shanna Lundy MS, Chad Eriksen BA and Beth K. 2007,** Flaxseed: A Review of Health Benefits, *Pennington Nutrition N°5, 4p*

182.   **Hermier D, Morise A, Ferezou J, Riottot, Fenart E and Weil P. 2004,** Influence of the form of lipid intake from flaxseed on cholesterol metabolism in hamsters. Oleaginous, Fatty substances, Lipid 11:230-236

183.   **Hillyer EV and Quesenberry KE.1997,** Dermatologic diseases In: Hillyer EV, Quesenberry KE, (Eds): Ferrets, Rabbits and Rodents, *Clinical Medicine and Surgery WB Saunders Company, Philadelphia, 432 pp, 212-213*

184.   **Hutchings, A.H. Scott, G. Lewis and A. Cunningham**, 1996, Zulu Medicinal plants: An inventory, (University of Natal Press, Pietermaritzburg)

185.   **Hutchins AM, Martini MC, Olson BA,Thomas W and Slavin JL. 2001,** Flaxseed consumption influences endogenous hormone concentrations in postmenopausal women, *Nutr Cancer* **39**(1):58-65, International Journal of Innovative Drug Discover ,4 (1):22-24

186.   **Hutchins AM and Slavin JL. 2003,** Effects of flaxseed on sex hormone metabolism. *In: Thompson LU, Cunnane SC, editors. Flaxseed in human nutrition. 2nd ed. Champaign, Ill: A American Oil Chemical Society Press. p 126-49.*

187.   **Iserin P. 2001,** Encyclopedie des plantes medicinales, identification, preparation, soin, 2$^{\wedge me}$ edition Ed Larousse/ VUEF, pp13- 16, p250, pp291-296

188.   **Jain DK, Patni P, Varghese D and BalekarN.2006,** Formulation and evaluation of herbal hair oil for alopecia management, *Planta India.* **2** *(3) :27- 30*

189.   **Janbaz KH and Gilani AH.1995,** Evaluation of the protective potential of Artemisia maritima extraction acetaminophen- and CCL4-induced liver damage, *Journal of Ethnopharmacology* **47***, 43-47*

190.   **Jaworsky C, Kligman AM and Murphy GF.1992,** Characterisation of inflammatory infiltrates in male pattern alopecia: Implication for pathogenesis. BR, *J. Dermatol* **127**: 239-246

191.   **Jhala Amit J and Hall LM.2010,** Flax (*Linum usitatissimum* L.): Current Uses and Future Applications: Australian *Journal of basic and Applied Sciences* 4(9): 4304-4312

192.   **Jonston DE.1993,** Thermal injuries. Deseases mechanisms in small animal surgery, 2$^{:m:}$ *Ed., Lea and Fibiger. Philadephia, 170-177*

193.   **Joucdar S. 1993,** La reparation esthetique des sequelles de brulures severes du cou. *Annals of the Mediterranean Burns Club, 6:33-40*

194.   **Kabarinta, K D A. 2010,** Healing properties of *Opilia celtidifolia* leaves. These of State Doctor in Pharmacy. Universite de Bamako. Faculte de Medecine de

Pharmacie et d'Odonto-Stomatologie. Mali. P109

195. **Kaddour MN et Haouem MS.2010,** Traitement de la brulure experimentale par un mélange de beurre frais et poudre de feuille de ronces, *Memoire en vue de l'obtention de diplome de docteure veterinaire. Universite Mentouri Constantine*, 102p

196. **Kaithwas G, Mukerjee A, Kumar P, Majumdar DK 2011,** Linum usitatissimum (linseed/flaxseed) fixed oil: antimicrobial activity and efficacy in bovine mastitis, InflammoPharmacology. 19: 45-52

197. **Kaithwas G, Mukherjee A, Chaurasia AK, Majumdar DK. 2011,** Antiinflammatory, analgesic and antipyretic activities of Linum usitatissimum L. (flaxseed/linseed) fixed oil, *Indian J. Exp. Biol 49:932-938*

198. **Kamath J.V., A.C. Rana and A.R. Chowdhury. 2003,** Pro-healing effect of *Cinnamomum zeylanicum* bark, *Phytotherapy research* 17: 970-972

199. **Kamimura A, Takahashi T. 2002,** Cutaneous biology procyanidin b-2, extracted from apples, promotes hair growth: a laboratory study, *British Journal of Dermatology 146:41-51*

200. **Kang-Bong S, Ja-Seon Y, Dang-Young K, Jae-Hwang J, Eun-Young K, Sang-Yoon N, Young-Won Y, Jong-Soo K and Beom-Jun L.2011,** Effects of Herbal Extracts on Hair Growth Promotion in Experimental Animal Mode. *Journal of Biomedical Research 12 (2): 113-120*

201. **Kaufman KD, Olsen EA, Whiting D, Savin R, Devillez R, Bergfeld W, Price VH, Van Neste D, Roberts JL, Hordinsky M, Shapiro J, Binkowitz B and Gormley GJ. 1998,** Finasteride in the treatment of men with androgenetic alopecia. finasteride male pattern hair loss study group, *J. AM. ACAD. Dermatol 39:578-589*

202. **Kerharo J, Adam JG. 1974,** La Pharmacopee Senegalaise Traditionnelle, *Plantes Medicinales et Toxiques.* Edn. Vigot Freres; 1011p

203. **Kierszenbaum. 2002,** Histology and Cell Biology, An Introduction to Anatomical Pathology, *Second Edition. P 300-314*

204. **Kim H and Choi H.2005,** Stimulation of acyl-coA oxidase by a-linolenic acid rich parilla oil lowers plasma tricylglycerol level in rats, *Life Sci 77: 1293-1306*

205. **Kobayashi N, Suzuki, Koide C, Suzuki T, Matsuda H and Kubo M.1993,** Effect of leaves of *Ginkgo biloba* on hair growth in C 3Hstrain mice, *Takagala Zasshi 113(10): 718-24*

206. **Kohler C. 2011,** External teguments or tegumentary apparatus, Course, de *College universitaire et hospitalier des histologistes, embryologistes, cytologistes et cytogeneticiens (CHEC) Universite Medicale Virtuelle Francophone.* Updated : 01/07/2012

207. **Kouba M, Benatmane F, Blochet JE, Mourot J.2008,** Effect of a linseed diet on lipid oxidation fatty acid composition of muscle, perirenal fat and raw and cooked rabbit, *Meat. Sci 80: 829-834*

208. **Kubena LF, Harvey RB, Huff WE, Elissalde MH, Yersin AG, Phillips TD and Rottinghaus GE. 1993,** Efficacy of hydrated sodium calcium aluminosilicate to reduce the toxicity of aflatoxin and diacetoxyscirpenol, *Journal of Poultry Sciences 72: 51-59*

209. **Kumar B, Vijayakumar M, Govindarajan R, Pushpangadan P. 2007,**

Ethnopharmacological approaches to wound Healing. Exploring medicinal plants of India, *Journal of Ethnopharmacolgy (114): 103-113.*

210.   **Kumar M.S., R. Sripriya, H.V. Raghavan, P.K. Sehgal. 2006,** Wound healing potential of *Cassia fistula* on infected Albino rat Model, *Journal of Surgical Research* 131: 283-289

211.   **Kumara Swamy H.M., V. Krishna, K. Shankarmurthy, B. Abdul Rahiman, K.L. Mankani, K.M. Mahadevan, B.G. Harish, H. Raja Naika (2007),** Wound healing activity of embelin isolated from the ethanol extract of leaves of *Embelia ribes* Burn, *Journal of Ethnopharmacology* 109: 529-534

212.   **Labrune HJ, Reinhardt CD, Dikeman ME, Drouillard JS.2008,** Effects of grain processing and dietary lipid source on performance, carcass characteristics, plasma fatty acids, and sensory properties of steaks from finishing cattle, *Journal of Animal Science 86(1):167-172*

213.   **Lachgar S, Charveron M, Gall Y and Bonafe JL. 1998,** Minoxidil upregulates the expression of vascular endothelial growth factor in human hair dermal papilla cells,BR. *J. Dermatol* (138): 407-411

214.   **Lanszki J, Thebault R, Allain D, Szendro Z and Eiben C. 2001,** The effects of melatonin treatment on wool production and hair follicle cycle in angora rabbits, *Animal.Res 50:79-89*

215.   **Laplante A. 2002,** Mecanismes de reepithelialisation des plaies cutanees : expression des proteines de stress chez la souris et analyse a l'aide d'un nouveau modele tridimensionnel humain developpe par genie tissulaire, These de doctorat en Medecine Experimentale, *Collection Memoires et theses electroniques. Universite LAVAL* , 230p

216.   **Larrey D.2005,** Hepato toxicite de la phytotherapie, *Formation Medicale Continue. SNFGE. Paris 3 April*

217.   **Latarjet J, Foyatier JL and Tchattirian E. 1992,** Brulures: etiologie, physiopathologie, diagnostic, principes du traitement precoce. *Rev Prat 42(12) :1565 -1572*

218.   **Le Bever H. 2009,** Les brulures etendues. (HIA Percy, Clamart) Capacite de Medecine d'Urgence : *1A Seminars 30 et 31mars 2009. SAMU de Paris*

219.   **Lebas F, Condert P, Rochambeau H and Thiebault RG.1996,** Le lapin elevage et pathologie, *Rome collection FAO, 227p*

220.   **Lebas F.2010,** Influence de l'alimentation sur les performances des lapins, *Seminaire Tunis 9 decembre2010.http //cuniculture.info/docs/elevage/profess- 04- Besoin.htm*

221.   **Lefort R. 2011,** Genodermatoses et dermatoses hereditaires chez le chat, *These pour obtenir le grade de docteur veterinaire. L'universite CLAUDE- BERNARD - LYON I (Medecine - Pharmacie) 92p*

222.   **Lehmann H. 2013,** The herbal medicine in Europe: status, registration, controls. *These de docteur en es Sciences Pharmaceutiques. University of Strasbourg Faculty of Pharmacy. 341P*

223.   **Lengani A, Lambouado FLB, Innocent PGB and Nikiema JB.2009,** Traditional medicine and kidney diseases in Burkina Faso. Nephrol ther, doi:10.1016/j.nephro.2009.07.11 . Accessed on 06/09/12

224.   **Leonhardt H.2001,** Histologie, Zytologie und Mikroanatomie des Menschen,

in Physiology of the skin II, *P. Pugliese, Editor, Allured Publishing Corporation*

225.   **Li WL, Zheng HC, Bukuru J, De Kimpeb N. 2004,** Natural medicines used in the traditional Chinese medical system for therapy of diabetes mellitus, *Journal of Ethnopharmacology 92:1 - 21*

226.   **Li M, Marubayashi A, Nakaya Y, Fukui K and Arase S.2001,** Minoxidil-induced hair growth is mediated by adenosine in cultured dermal papilla cells: Possible involvement of sulfonylurea receptor 2b as a target of minoxidil, *Journal of. Investigatives. Dermatology. 117:1594-1600.83*

227.   **Li S.1992,** In: Miyashita, S. (Ed.), Bencao-gangmu, reprint ed. Orient Publishing Co. Ltd, Osaka, pp. 579-580

228.   **Liang T and Liao S.1997,** Growth suppression of hamster flank organs by topical application of c-linolenic and other fatty acid inhibitors of 5a-reductase, *Journal of Investigative Dermatology* (1997) **109**, 152-157; doi:10.1111/1523-1747.ep12319203

229.   **Linnaeus C. 1857,** Species Plantarum, *The Royal Society of London, London, UK, pp: 300*

230.   **Loden, M., Andersson, AC. 1996,** Effect of topically applied lipids on surfactant-irritated skin,British Journal of Dermatology. 134(2) : 215-220

231.   **Lodhi S., R. Singh Pawer, A. Pal Jai, A.K. Singhai (2006),** Wound healing potential of *Tephrosia purpurea* (Linn.) Pers. in rats, *Journal of Ethnopharmacology* 108: 204-210

232.   **Luelmo -Aguilar J, M.S Santandreu. 2004.** Folliculitis: Recognition and management. *American Journal of* Clinics Dermatology 5: 301-310

233.   **Maameri Z, Beroual K, Djerrou Z, Habibatni S, Benlaksira B, Serrakta A, Mansour-Djaalab H, Kahlouche-Riachi F, Bachtari K and Hamdi Pacha Y.2012,** Preliminary study to assess cicatrizing activity of honey and *Pistacia lentiscus* fatty oil mixture on experimental burns in rabbits, *International. Journal of.Medinal and Aromatics. Plants* 3(4): 476-480

234.   **Maameri- Habibatni Z. 2014,** *Pistacia lentiscus L.:* Evaluation pharmacotoxicologique, *These in view of obtaining the diploma of Doctorat en Sciences. Option : Pharmacologie Toxicologie Universite de Constantine. Algerie. 138p*

235.   **MacKay, D., Miller, A.L., 2003,** Nutritional Support for Wound Healing. Alternative Medicine Review. 8 (4), 359-377

236.   **Maddock TD, Bauer ML, Koch KB, Anderson VL, Maddock RJ, Barcelo-Coblijn G, Murphy EJ and Lardy GP.2006,** Effect of processing flax in beef feedlot diets on performance, carcass characteristics, and trained sensory panel ratings1, *Journal of Animal Science 84 (6):*1544-1551

237.   **Majtan J, Kumar P, Majtan T, Walls AF, Khudiny J.2010,** Effect of honey and its major royal jelly .protein 1 on cytokine and MMP-9 mRNA transcripts in human keratinocytes, *Experimental Dermatology 19(8) : 19, 73-79*

238.   **Majunder, P., 2010,** Preliminary phytochemical and wound healing activity of *Zyziphus oenoplia.* Master of Pharmacy; Department of Pharmacognosy. Karnataka. India

239.   **Malnoux B.1991,** Troubles endocriniens et hyperpigmentation de la peau chez le chien (etude de 478 cas cliniques), *These de doctorat vétérinaire, Faculte de*

medecine, Nantes, 94p

240. **Manjeshwar Shrinath B, Ganesh Chandra J, Jagadish NU and Manjeshwar Poona B.2004,** The evaluation of the acute toxicity and long term safety of hydrialcoholic extract of Sapthaparna (*Alstonia scholaris*) in mice and rats, *Toxicology Letters* **151**: *317-326*

241. **Mansour-Djaalab H, Kahlouche-Riachi F, Djerrou Z, Serakta- Delmi A, Hamimed S, Trifa W, Djaalab I, Hamdi-Pacha Y, Maotti R and Musarelle P. 2012,** *In vitro* evaluation of antifungal effects of *Lawsonia inermis, Pistacia lentiscus* and *Juglans regia, International. Journal of Medicinal and. Aromatics. Plants* **2**(2): 263-268

242. **Mantzioris E, James MJ, Gibson RA and Cleland LG. 1995,** Nutritional attributes of dietary flaxseed oil, *American Journal of Clinical Nutrition* **62**(4): 841

243. **Mantzioris E, James MJ, Gibson RA and Cleland LG.1994,** Dietary substitution with an alpha-linolenic acid-rich vegetable oil increases eicosapentaenoic acid concentrations in tissues, *American Journal Clinical* **Nutrition***59(6):1304-1309*

244. **Marieb EN. 1993,** Anatomie et physiologie humaines, *Editions du Renouveau Pedagogique Inc, Quebec, 192p*

245. **Marieb EN.2005,** Human anatomy and physiology, sixth edition, *Pearson Education, France, 212p*

246. **Martin A. 1996,** The use of antioxidants in healing, *Dermatologic Surgery*. 22: 156-160

247. **Martin A. 2001,** Apports nutritionnels conseillilles pour la population frangaise, *Tec et Doc, 3rd edition, Paris.*

248. **Martin C, H Dubbroeucq, D Micol, J Agabriel, M Doreau 2007,** Methane output from beef cattle fed different high-concentrate diets, *Annual Conference of the British Society of Animal Science, 2-4 April Dublin p 46*

249. **Martin P. 1997,** Wound healing-aiming for perfect skin regeneration, Science (276), 75-81

250. **Masonc L K.1993,** Treatment of contaminated wounds, including wounds of the abdomen and thorax, *In HARARI, J.: Surgical complications and wound healing in the small animal practice. Philadelphia, Saunders, W.B., 1993, 33-62*

251. **Masson-Meyers DS , Enwemeka CS, Bumah VV, Andrade TAM, Cashin SE, Frade MAC 2013,** Antimicrobial effects of *Copaifera langsdorffli oleoresin* in infected rat wounds, International Journal of Applied Microbiology Science; 2(3):9-20

252. **Maurette Jean-Marc, 2008,** Flaxseed oil, a fish oil challenger? Oleaginous, Corps gras, Lipides, (15) 4 :257-261

253. **Maurin L.2005,** Le porc modele animal de cicatrisation cutanee, *These de docteur veterinaire Universite Claude Bernard Lyon I (Medecine- Pharmacie) 138p*

254. **Mazza G and Oomah BD.1995,** Flaxseed, dietary fiber and cyanogens, *In: Cunnane S, Thompson LU (Eds) Flaxseed in human nutrition AOCS Press, Champaign, Illinois, pp. 56-81*

255. **McClellan JK and Markham A.1999,** Finesteride. A review of its use in male pattern hair loss, *Drugs 57(1):111 126*

256. **McDaniel JC, Belury M, Ahijevych K, Blakely W., (2008),** Omega-3 fatty acids effect on wound healing, Wound Repair Regen. 16(3): 337-45

257. **Mcelwee KJ, and Sinclair RD. 2008,** Hair physiology and its disorders, *Drug*

Discovery Today: Disease Mechanisms **5** *(2):163-71*

258. **Mcewan and Jenkinson D.1970,** The distribution of nerves, monoamineoxidase and cholinesterase in the skin of the guinea Pig, hamster, mouse, rabbit and rat, Research in Veterinary Science *II: 60-70*

259. **Mekroud A.2004,** La biochimie medicale en medicine veterinaire, *Les editions de l'universite de Constantine, 105p*

260. **Millam s, Bohus O and Anna P.2005,** Plant cell and biotechnology studies in *Linum usitatissimum* - A review, Plant Cell Tissue Organ Cult **82**: 93-103

261. **Millar WJ.1997,** Use of alternative health care practitioners by Canadians, Canadian *Journal of Public Health* **88**:154-8

262. **Mitz V.1994,** La cicatrisation dirigee, *Revue de praticien* **13**(*4):1743-1750*

263. **Monteiro Riviere NA, Stinson ALWL and Calhoun H. 1993,** Text book of veterinary histology, *4th edition, USA, Lea and febiger*

264. **Monteiro-Riviere NA.1998,** Integument, *In: Delmann HD, JA Eurell, (Eds): Text book of veterinary histology, lippincot Williams and Wilkine, Baltimore, Maryland, USA: 303-332.ISBN:978-0-7817-4148-4*

265. **Moore GPM, Jackson N, Issacs K, Brown G.1998,** Patter and morphogenesis in skin, *Journal of Theoretical Biology* **191**: *87:94*

266. **Morasso MI and Tomic M. 2005,** Epidermal stem cells: the cradle of epidermal determination, differentiation and wound healing, *Biology of the cell / under the auspices of the European Cell Biology Organization* **97**(*3):173-83*

267. **Moretti G, Rampini E and Rebora A.1976,** The hair cycle re-evaluated, International *Journal of Dermatology* **15**:277-285

268. **Morris, D.H. 2003,** Flax: A health and nutrition primer, *3rd ed, p.11 Winnipeg: Flax Council of Canada Downloaded from http://www.jitinc.com/flax/brochure02.pdf verified on 4/6/12*

269. **Morris, D.H. 2003,** Flax: A health and nutrition primer. 3rd ed, p.11 Winnipeg: Flax Council of Canada. Downloaded from http://www.jitinc.com/flax/brochure02.pdf. Accessed 4/6/12

270. **Moukal A. 2004,** The Argan tree, *Argania spinosa.L (skeels),* use therapeutics, cosmetics and food, *Phytotherapie* **5** *:135-141*

271. **Mourot J. 2008,** Modification de la qualite nutritionnelle des produits animaux, *3m journee CEREL, Rennes, 3 et 4 juillet, 14-23*

272. **Mourot J.2010,** How can we improve the nutritional quality of animal fats nutrition- sante (January- February), *Oleaginous,Corps gras,Lipides* **17**:*37- 42*

273. **Muir AD. 2006,** Flax lignans--analytical methods and how they influence our understanding of biological activity, *Journal of* Association of Official Analytical Chemists *International* **89**(4):1147-1157

274. **Muller GH and Kirk RW.1975,** Dermatology of small animals, *Edt: Vigots freres, 55-66, 133-1*

275. **Muller GH, Kirk RW, Scott DW. 2001,** Structure and function of the skin, *In Muller G.H, Kirk R.W, small animal dermatology Saunders (Ed): 1-70.99*

276. **Murty M, Kevin Bernardo NDB, Sc Sron Tam SJM and Sc Zimmerman M. 2012,** Adverse effects of natural health products in children: A practical guide to screening and reporting. Canadian Paediatric Surveillance Program Resources (3), 7p

277. **Narayan D, Indrajit K, Kar RB, Suresh K, Biswa KK, Asis B and Pallab KH.2012,** Free radical scavenging activity of *Castanopsis indicain* mediating hepatoprotective activity of carbon tetrachloride intoxicated rats. *Asian Pacific Journal of Tropical Biomedicin: S242-S251*

278. **Nelson GJ and Chamberlain G.1995,** The effect of dietary alphalinolenic Acid on blood lipids and lipoproteins in human, *In: Cunnane S, Thompson LU (Eds) Flaxseed in human nutrition. American Oil Chemists' Society Press, Champaign, Illinois, pp. 56-81*

279. **Nergard, C. S., 2005,** Immunomodulating pectic polymers, PhD thesis, Department of Pharmacognosy. University of Oslo, Norway, 80p

280. **Noli C.1999,** Structure and function of the skin and coat, *In: GUAGUERE E. and P. PRELAUD, Guide Pratique de Dermatologie Feline.(1999), Ed. Merial. Lyon*

281. **Noli, C, M. Welle, F. Scarampella F. Abramo, 2003,** Quantitative analysis of tryptase and chymase-containing mast cells in eosinophilic condition of cats. *Veterinary Pathology, 40, 219-221*

282. **Noli C. 2006,** Structure and physiology of the skin and coat, *In GUAGERE E, PRELAUD P. Guide pratique de dermatologie canine. Marial Kalianxis (Ed):17-30*

283. **Norwood OT. 2001,** Incidence of female androgenetic alopecia (female pattern alopecia), *Dermatol. Surg **27**:53-54*

284. **Norwood OT.1975;** Male-pattern baldness. Classification and incidence *South Med. J **68**:1359-1370*

285. **O'Neill, W., Sharyn McKee, Andrew F. Clarke 2002,** Flaxseed (Linum usitatissimum) supplementation associated with reduced skin test lesional area in horses with Culicoides hypersensitivity The Canadian Journal of Veterinary Research;66:272.277

286. **Ognik K, Czech A, Sembratowicz I, Laszzwska M. 2012,** Influence of linseed oil on selected parameters of blood and production performance of turkey hens, *Annales universitatis Mariae curie-skfodowska Lublin - Polonia **EE** (4): 76-83*

287. **Olivera- Martinez I, Viallet Jp and Michon F.2004,** The different steps of skin formation in vertebrates, International Journal of Developmental Biology 48:137-48

288. **Ono I, Tateshita T and Inoue M.1999,** Effects of a collagen matrix containing basic fibroblast growth factor on wound contraction, *J Biomed mater Res (Appl Biomater) **48**: 621-630*

289. **Oomah B. 2003,** Processing of flaxseed fiber,oil, protein, and lignin, *In:Thompson, L., Cunnane, S. Editores. Flaxseed in Human Nutrition. 2nd. Edn. Champaing, Illinois. 363-386*

290. **Oomah BD.2001,** Flaxseed as a functional food source. Journal of the Science of Food and Agricultural, *J. Sci. Food Agr* 81(9): 889-894

291. **Orhue NEJ, Nwanze EAC and Okafor A. 2005,** Serum total protein, albumin and globulin levels in Trypanosoma brucei-infected rabbits: Effect of orally administered *Scoparia dulcis, African Journal of Biotechnology 4 **(10)**: 11521155*

292. **Otberg N, Finner AM and Shapiro J.2007,** Androgenetic alopecia, *Endocrinol Metab Clin North Am 36:379-398in 95/ mcelwee kj. and sinclair rodney (2008)*

293. **Ouhayoun J. 1989,** La viande de lapin, composition de la fraction comestible

de la carcasse et des morceaux de decoupe, *Cunicole- science 5:1- 6*

294.   **Oznurlu Y, Celik I, Sur E, Telatar T and Ozparlak H .2009,** Comparative Skin Histology of the White New Zealand and Angora Rabbits: Histometrical and Immunohistochemical Evaluations, *Journal of Animal and Veterinary Advances* 8(9):1694-1701

295.   **Palazzi X. 2002,** Semiologie macroscopique et microscopique de la peau), *These de doctorat veterinaire, Universite Claude Bernard, Lyon, 76 p*

296.   **Palmeri, B., Glauco, G. and Palmeri, G. 1995,** Vitamin E added silicone gel sheets for treatment of hypertophic scars and keloids. *International Journal of Dermatology.* 34 : 506-509

297.   **Park J.E, Barbul. A. 2004,** Understanding the role of immune regulation in wound healing. American Journal of Surgery 187(S): 6-11

298.   **Patil SM, Sapkale GN, Surwase US and Bhombe BT. 2010,** Herbal medicines as an effective therapy in hair loss - a review, *Research Journal of Pharmaceutical, Biological and Chemical Sciences 2(1):773-781*

299.   **Patterson CA. 2006,** Bioactive compounds from flax. Canadian Healthy Ingredients, *Agriculture and Agri-Food Canada: 1-4*

300.   **Paus R and Cotsarelis G.1999,** Biology of the hair follicle, N Engl.*J.Med* **341**:491-497

301.   **Paus R, Stenn KS and Link RE. 1990,** Telogen skin contains an inhibitor of hair growth, *British Journal of Dermatology 122:777-784*

302.   **Paus R. 1998,** Principles of hair cycle control, Journal of Dermatology 25:793-802

303.   **Pavletic MM.2003,** The integument. In slatter D editor. Textbook of small animal surgery, *Third edition Philadelphia. W.B Saunder: 250-259*

304.   **Pavletic, M.M. (1985),** Introduction to wound healing and wound management, Process American Animal. Hospital Association: 655-663

305.   **Perumal Samy R., P. Gopalakrishnakone, M. Sarumathi, S. Ignacimuthu (2006),** Wound healing potential of *Tragia involucrate* extract in rats, *Fitoterapia* 77: 300-302

306.   **Peters EMJ, Handjiski B and Kuhlmann A. 2004,** Neurogenic inflammation in stress-induced termination of murine hair growth is promoted by nerve growth factor, *American Journal of Pathology, Vol. 165, No. 1,: 259-271*

307.   **Peterschmitt M. 2009,** L'Ambre chez le chat des forets, norvegienne, un Mystere Resolu, *Memoire de docteur Veterinaire, Ecole nationale veterinaire de Lyon. Universite Claude Bernard, Lyon I (Medecine- pharmacie). 218p*

308.   **Pierard-Franchimont C and Pierard GE.2001,** Teloptosis, a turning point in hair shedding biorhythms, *Dermatology 203 :115-117*

309.   **Pillon F. 2013,** Les alopecies medicamenteuses, transitoires mais invalidantes, *Actualites Pharmaceutiques 522: 46-47*

310.   **Pooja S, Banerjee M, Sharma R and Kumar N. 2009,** Preparation, evaluation and hair growth stimulating activity of herbal hair oil,*Journal of Chemical and Pharmaceutical Research 1*(1): 261-267

311.   **Pradhan R, Meda V, Rout P, Naik S and Dalai A. 2010,** Supercritical CO2 extraction of fatty oil from flaxseed and comparison with screw press expression and solvent extraction processes. *Journal of Food Engineering 98(4): 393-397*

312.   **Prasad A, Ritesh K, Harini R, Nalini Krishnananda P.2012,** *A Case of Flax Seed Induced: Rhabdomyolysis. Journal of Clinical and Diagnostic Research 6(10): 1770-1771*

313.   **Prasad K. 2000,** Oxidative stress as a mechanism of diabetes in diabetic BB prone rats: Effect of secoisolariciresinol diglucoside (SDG) isolated from flaxseed, *Molecular and* Cellular Biochemistry *209:89-96*

314.   **Prasad K.1997,** Dietary flax seed in prevention of hypercholesterolemic atherosclerosis. *Atherosclerosis 7-11132 (1):69-76*

315.   **Price VH. 1999,** Treatment of hair loss, *New England Journal of Medicine 341:964-973.*

316.   **Priya K.S., A. Gnanamani, N. Radhakrichnan, M. Babu (2002),** Healing potential of *Datura alba* on burn wounds in albino rats, *Journal of Ethnipharmacology* 83: 193-199

317.   **Probst CW. et al. 1984,** The surgical management of a large thermal burn in a dog, *Journal of the American Animal Hospital Association.* 20, 45-49

318.   **Prost-Squarcioni, C., (2006),** Histology of the skin and hair follicles, *Medecine/Sciences 22: 131-137*

319.   **Pu ZB, Wang CC, Liu HB, Zhou LG, Chao CR, Sang ZX, Dong F, Ge Jl. 1999,** Experimental study on the effect of Moist Exposed Burn Therapy/Moist. Exposed Burn Ointment on burn wound water evaporation. The Chinese Journal of Burns Wounds and Surface Ulcers, February. 11(1): 1-3

320.   **Purwal L, Surya-prakash BN, Gupta and Milind SP. 2008,** Development and evaluation of herbal, formulations for hair growth, *E-Journal of Chemistry 1(5): 34-38*

321.   **Quinn MJ, Moore ES, Thomson DU, Depenbusch BE, May ML, Higgins JJ, Carter JF and Drouillard JS. 2008,** The effect of feeding flaxseed during the receiving period on morbidity, mortality, performance, and carcass characteristics of heifers,*Journal of Animal Science 86 (11): 3054-3061*

322.   **Quinton JF. 2003,** Nouveaux animaux de Compagnie : *Peties Mamiferes, Ed: Maloine, p. 66*

323.   **Radi N. 2003,** L'Arganier : arbre de sud-ouest Marocain ; en peril ; a proteger, *These pour le diplome d'etat de Docteur en pharmacie Universite de NANTES. Faculte de pharmacie,* 59p

324.   **Rafieian-kopaei M.2013,** Medicinal plants for renal injury prevention, *Journal of Renal Injury Prevention 2(2): 63-65*

325.   **Randall VA, Thornton MJ, Hamada K, Redfern CP, Nutbrown M and Ebling FJ. 1991,** Messenger AG. Androgens and the hair follicle. Cultured human dermal papilla cells as a model system. *Annals of New York Academy of Science 642: 355-375.*

326.   **Randall VA, Thornton MJ and Hamada K.1992,** Messenger AG. Mechanism of androgen action in cultured dermal papilla cells derived from human hair follicles with varying responses to androgens in vivo. *Journal of Investigative Dermatology 98:86S-91S*

327.   **Ravat FJ, Peslages PP and Fontaine NM .2011,** Sens La brulure : une pathologie inflammatoire, *Pathologie biologie 59(3) : e63-e72*

328.   **Rebora A, Guarrera M. 2002,** Kenogen. A new phase of the hair cycle, *Dermatology 205, (2):108-110*

329.   **Remdios A.1999,** Complication of wound healing, *In fowlerD, williams, J, M,. britch small animal veterinary association 5: 137-143*

330.   **Renouard S. 2011,** Regulation transcriptionnelle de la biosynthese des lignanes du lin (*Linum usitatissimum* et *Linum flavum*) et amelioration de lignane extraction, *These de Docteur de l'Université d'Orleans, Ecole doctorale sciences et technologies, Pole universite, Centre Val de Loire, 231p*

331.   **Reygane P. (2009),** Diffuse female alopecia: no resignation, *12es advancee en gynecologie et obstetrique CAP 15 Paris .Centre Sabouraud*

332.   **Rho SS, Chang Deok K, Min-Ho L, Seong-Lok H, Moon-Jeong R and Yeo-Kyeong Y.2002,** The hair growth promoting effect of *Sophora flaavescens* extract and its molecular regulation, *Journal of Dermatological Science 30:4349*

333.   **Rho SS, Su-Jin P, Seong-Lok H, Min-Ho L, Chang Deok K, In-Ho L, Sug-Youn C and Moon-Jeong R.2005,** The hair growth promoting effect of Asiasari radix extract and its molecular regulation, *Journal of Dermatological Science 38: 89-97*

334.   **Ricard SE, Orcheson LJ, Seidl MM, Lyengi L, Fong HH and Thompson LU.1996,** Dose-dependent production of mammalian lignans in rats and in vitro from the purified precursor secoisolariciresinol diglycoside *Flaxseed. Journal of Nutrition 126(8): 2012-2019.*

335.   **Ricard SE and Thompson LU.1997,** Phytoestrogens and lignans: effects on reproduction and chronic disease, *In: Antinutrients and Phytochemicals in Food (Shahidi, F., ed.), pp. 273-293. American Chemical Society, Washington, DC*

336.   **Richet G. 1988,** Nephrology, *Editions Ellipes/Aupelf, p361*

337.   **Robert.1982,** Identification des poils des mammiferes domestiques.*These de doctorat veterinaire, Universite Paul Sabatier, Toulouse, 67p*

338.   **Roberto Chiej.1982 ,** Les plantes medicinales; *Guide vert; Solar: Paris, 500p*

339.   **Rochambeau H and Vrillon IL.1985,** Factors of variation of the quality of the fur and of the weight productivity in the domestic rabbit, *Annale de Zootechie 34: 49-79*

340.   **Rondia P, Delmotte C, Dehareng F, Maene D, Toussaint JF and Bertiaux-Thill N. 2003,** Incidence d'un apport en graines de lin chez la brebis et l'agneau sur les performances et le profil en acides gras de la viande d'agneaux eleves en bergerie ou en paturage, *Rencontre, Recherche, Ruminants 10 : 227-230*

341.   **Rose RL and Hodgson E. 2004,** Metabolism of Toxicants pp 111-149 A *Textbook of Modern Toxicology, Third Edition, edited by Ernest Hodgson . Copyright John Wiley & Sons, Inc*

342.   **Rossant A. 2011,** Honey, a complex compound with surprising properties. *These: for the diploma of state of doctor in pharmacy faculty of pharmacy. University of Limoges, 113p*

343.   **Rougeot J et Thebault RG.1983,** Variation saisonniere de la composition et de la structure du pelage : exemple de la toison du lapin angora, *Annale de Zootechnie 32 : 287-314*

344.   **Roy RK, Mayank T, Dixit VK. 2008,** Hair growth promoting activity of eclipta alba in male albino rats, Archives of Dermatological Research *300:357-364*

345.   **Rubilar M, Gutierrez C, Vedugo M, Shene C and Sineiro J.2010,** Flaxseed as a source of functional ingredients. *Journal of soil Science, Plant Nutrition 10 (3): 373-377*

346.   **Ruckebusch Y. 1981,** Physiologique pharmacologique therapeutique

animales, *2eme edition Maloine SA paris, p611.*

347. **Rupniak NM and Kramer MS.1999,** Discovery of the antidepressant and antiemetic efficacy of substance P receptor (NK1) antagonists, *Trends Pharmacol Sci* **20:485-490.**

348. **Sadaf F., R. Saleem, M. Ahmed, A. Syed Iqbal, L. Navaidul-Zafar. 2006,** Healing potential of cream containing extract of *Sphaeranthus indicus* on dermal wounds in Guinea pigs, *Journal of Ethnopharmacology* 107: 161-163

349. **Sandford JC.1979,** The domestic rabbit, 3rd edition. London Granada publishing, 258p

350. **Sandhya.S , Sai Kumar.P, Vinod K.R, David Banji, Kumar K. 2011,** Plants as potent anti-diabetic and wound healing agents: A review, *Hygeia Journal for Drugs and Medicines 3 (1):11-19*

351. **Sarkhail P, Rahmanipour S, Fadyevatan S, Mohammadirad A, Dehghan G, Amin G, Shafiee A and Abdollahi M.2007,** Antidiabetic effect of *Phlomis anisodonta*: Effects on hepatic cells lipid peroxidation and antioxidant enzymes in experimental diabetes, *Pharmacological Research, 56:261 - 266*

352. **Savin RC and Atton AV.1993,** Minoxidil: update on its clinical role, Dermatologic Clinics **11**: 55-64

353. **Schaffer A and Mednche N. 2004,** Anatomie physiologie biologie, second edition, Maloine, pp 154-158

354. **Scohier PE.2000,** Treatment of chronic skin wounds in a horse with honey (clinical case), les Grandes Plaines, Centre Veterinaire des Grandes Plaines Froidchapelle - Belgium, 5p

355. **Scott DW, Miller WH and Griffin CE.1995,** Small Animal Dermatology, *MULLER G, Kirk's (Ed). 5th edition. WB SAUNDERS Co, Philadelphia, 2-54 ET 1127-1173*

356. **Seigue A.1985,** La foret circummediterraneenne et ses problemes. Maisonneuve et La rose *In foret mediterraneenne, t. VII, no 2, 141-142*

357. **Serakta Delmi M. (1999),** Effet cicatrisantes des huiles de genevrier oxycedre, pin d'Alep, cedre d'atlas sur les brulures experimentales, *Diplome de magistere, medicine vétérinaire. Universite Constantine 95p. Algeria*

358. **Shanmuga Priya KS, Gnanamani A, Radhakrishnan N, Babu M. 2002,** Healing potential of *Datura alba* on burn wounds in albino rats. Journal of Ethnopharmacology 83: 193-199

359. **Sharma SB, Nasir A, Prabhu KM and Murthy PS. 2006,** Antihyperglycemic effect of 300 the fruit-pulp of *Eugenia jambolana* in experimental diabetes mellitus, *Journal of Ethnopharmacology 104: 367-373*

360. **Shimizu M, Kobayashi Y, Suzuki M, Satsu H and Miyamoto Y.2000,** Regulation of intestinal glucose transport by tea catechins, *Biofactors 13: 61 - 65*

361. **Shipra Gupta, Sharmaa SB, Kumar Bansalb S and Prabhua KM.2009,** Antihyperglycemic and hypolipidemic activity of aqueous extract of *Cassia auriculata* L. leaves in experimental diabetes. *Journal of Ethnopharmacology 123(3):499-503. doi: 10.1016/j.jep.2009.02.019*

362. **Shivhare Y, Prashant S, Shurkia S, Patel JR, (2014a),** Potentials of medicinal plants as wound healers: A review .Research Journal of Pharmacognosy and Phytochemistry 6 (1):41-43

363. **Shivhare*, Y., J.R. Patel, Prashant Soni, (2014b),** Healing efficacy of *trichosanthes dioica* roxb on dead space wounds, *International Journal of Innovative Drug discovery, 4: Vol 4 / Issue 1 :22-24.*

364. **Sifour, M., Ouled-Hadddar, H., Ouitas, L., Kerfa, A., 2012,** Burn Healing Activity of Aqueous Extract of *Atractylis gummifera. International Seminar: Cancer, cellular stress and bioactive substances. Jijel, 23-24 Sep. Algeria. 7174*

365. **Siguel EN.1994,** Essential and trans fatty acid metabolism in health and disease. *Comprehensive Therapy 20(9):500-510*

366. **Silvetti AN. 1981,** An effective method of treating long enduring wounds ulcers by tropical applications of solutions of nutrients, *Journal of Dermatology, Surgery and Oncology 7(6): 501-508*

367. **Sinclair R.1998,** Male pattern androgenetic alopecia, *British Medical Journal 317:865-869*

368. **Singer, A.J., Clark, R.A., 1999,** Cutaneous wound healing. *New England Journal of Medicine 341 (10): 738-746*

369. **Singh M., R. Govindarajan, V. Nath, A.K. Singh Rawat, S. Mehrotra. 2006,** Antimicrobial, wound healing and antioxidant activity of *Plagiochasma appendiculatum* Lehm. And Lind, *Journal of Ethnopharmacology* 107: 67-72

370. **Singh S and Majumdar DK. 1997,** Evaluation of anti-inflammatory activity of fatty acids of *Ocimum sanctum* fixed oil. Indian, *Journal of Experimental Biology 35:380-383*

371. **Soma T, Ogo M, Suzuki J, Takahachi T and Hibino T. 1998,** Analysis of apoptotic cell death in human hair follicles in vivo and vitro, *Journal of Investigative Dermatology* **111**: 948-954

372. **Sperling LC. 1991** , Hair anatomy for the clinician. *Journal of American Academy of Dermatology* 25,1(1): 1-17

373. **Spindler JR.1988,** The safety of topical minoxidil solution in the treatment of pattern baldness: The results of a 27-center trial, *Clin Dermatol* **6***: 200-212*

374. **Srivastava P and Durgaprasad S.2008,** Burn wound healing property of *Cocos nucifera*: An appraisal. I, *Indian Journal of Pharmacology 40* **(4)** *:144- 146*

375. **Stenn KS and Paus R. 2001,** Controls of hair follicle cycling. *Physiological Reviews81(1):450-481*

376. **Stoll AL, Locke CA, Marangell LB and Severus WE. 1999,** Omega-3 fatty acids and bipolar disorder: a review, *Prostaglandins Leukot Essent Fatty Acids* **60**(5-6):329-337

377. **Suguna L., P. Sivakumar and G. Chandrakasan. 1996,** Effects of *Centella asiatica* extract on dermal wound healing in rats, *Indian Journal of Experimental Biology* 34: 1208-1211

378. **Suguna L., S. Singh, P. Sivakumar, P. Sampath and G. Chandrakasan, 2002,** Influence of *Terminalia chebulla* on dermal wound healing in rats, *Phytother Research 16: 227-231*

379. **Sumitra M., P. Manikandan and L. Suguna. 2005,** Effect of *Butea monosperma* on dermal wound healing in rats, *The International Journal of Biochemistry & Cell Biology* 37: 566-573

380. **Sundberg A, Appelkwist EL, Dallner G and Nilsson R. 1994,** Glutathione transferase in the urine: sensitive methods for detection of kidney damage induced

by nephrotoxic agents in humans, *Environ Health Perspect* **102**: 293296

381.	**Suntar, I., Ufuk Koca, Hikmet Keles_a ,Esra Kupeli Akkol, 2011,** Wound healing activity of *Rubus sanctus* schreber (rosaceae): preclinical study in animal models. Evidence-Based Complementary and Alternative Medicine, Article ID 816156. doi:10.1093/ecam/nep137: 1-6

382.	**Suraja R, Rejitha G, Sunilson JJ and Anandarjagopal K.2009,** In vivo hair growth activity of Prunus dulcis seeds in rats, Biology and Medicine *1 (4): 3438*

383.	**Swaim SF, Vaughn DM and Kincaid SA. 1990,** Effects of locally injected medications on healing of pad wounds in dogs, *American journal of veterinary* **57**: *394-399*

384.	**Swain, S.K., Rangacharyulu, P.V., Sarkar,S., K.M.Das.1996,** Effect of a probiotic supplementation on growth, nutrient utilization and carcass composition in mrigal fry, *Aquaculture.4:29-35*

385.	**Swaim, S.F., Henderson, R.A., 1997,** wound dressing materials and topical medication, *Small Animal Wound Management 2 Ed .William and wilkins editors. Baltimore, 53-85*

386.	**Tahraoui A, Zafar H, Israil I, Baddial Y.2010,** Acut and sub-chronic toxicity of lyophilized aqueous extract of *Centaurium erythraea* in rodents, *Journal of Ethnopharmacology* **132**:*48-55*

387.	**Tan KP, Chen J, Ward WE and Thompson LU. 2004,** Mammary gland morphogenesis is enhanced by exposure to flaxseed or its major lignan during suckling in rats, *Experimental Biology and Medicine* **229**:*147-57*

388.	**Thebaul RG.1977,** Le lapin Angora, developpement post natal de sa toison, variation saisonniere de la production de poil, *Memoire en vue de l'obtention du diplome d'ingenieur DEP. Conservatoire National des Arts et Metier. Paris. 111p.*

389.	**Thibaut S, Gaillard O, Bouhanna P.2005,** Human hair shape is pro: grammed from the bulb, *Journal of Dermatology (4)152: 632- 8*

390.	**Thompson LU. 2003,** Flaxseed in human nutrition, *2nd Edition, AOCS Press, Champaign, Illinois, 458 p*

391.	**Thorburn GD,Casey BH and Molyneux GS.2012,** Distribution of Blood Flow within the Skin of the Rabbit with Particular Reference to Hair growth, *Circulation Research* **1966** *(18):650-659*

392.	**Tomczak C.(2010),** Use of honey in the treatment of jokes, *Memoire de docteur veterinaire. Ecole veterinaire de Lyon* 187p

393.	**Tomoya T, Toshikazu K, Atsuhiro H, Yoshiharu Y.1999,** Procyanidin oligomers selectively and intensively promote proliferation of mouse hair epithelial cells in vivo, *Society for investigative Dermatology* **113**: *310-316*

394.	**Tonks AJ, Cooper RA, Jones KP, Blair S, Parton J, Tonks A.2003,** Honey stimulates inflammatory cytokine production from monocytes,*Cytokine* **21**(5): 242-247

395.	**Trueb RM. 2009,** Chemotherapy-induced alopecia, Seminars in Cutaneous Medicine and Surgery **28**:*11-14*

396.	**Trueb RM.2002,** Molecular mechanisms of androgenetic alopecia, *Experimental Gerontology* **37**:*981-990*

397.	**Tsuboi R.1997,** Growth factors and hair growth, *Korean Journal of Investigative Dermatology* **4**:*103-108*

398.   **Uno H and Kurata S.1993,** Chemical agents and peptides affect hair growth, *Journal of Investigative Dermatology **101:** 143-147*

399.   **Upadhyay S, Dixit V, Ghosh K, AK, Singh V, 2012a,** Effect of petroleum ether and ethanol fractions of seeds of Abrus precatorius on androgenic alopecia. Revista. Brasileira Farmacognosia (Brazilian Journal of Pharmacognosy), 22: 359-363.

400.   **Upadhyay S, Ashoke, Ghosh K, Vijender, Singh. 2012b,** Hair growth promoting activity of petroleum ether root extract of glycyrrhiza glabra l (fabaceae) in female rats. *Tropical Journal of Pharmaceutical Research; **11** (5): 753-758*

401.   **Upadhyay S, Ghosh A K, Singh V. 2014,** Inefficiency of ethanolic extract of *Glycyrrhiza glabra* and *Ziziphus mauritiana* roots on androgenic alopecia, *Journal of Pharmaceuticale Negative Results 5:25-8*

402.   **Vaisey-Genser M and Morris DH.2003,** Introduction: history of the cultivation and uses of flaxseed, *In Muir, A. D. and Westcott, N. D. (Eds). Flax: The genus Linum. p. 1-2. London: Taylor & Francis*

403.   **Van Hellement J. 1986,** Compendium of phytotherapy. Brussels, Belgium: Association Pharmaceutique Belge, 300-1

404.   **Venkateswaran S, Pari L, Viswanathan P and Menon V.1995,** Protective effect of livex, an herbal formulation against erythromycin estolate induced hepatotoxicity in rats, *Journal of Ethnopharmacology **57:** 161-167*

405.   ***Verola O. (2006),*** Anatomo-pathological aspects of wound healing, Cicatrisation.info : le livre "www.cicatrisation.info", consulted 06/06/2013

406.   **Viala A and Botta A. 2007,** Toxicology, *2m^e edition. Ed: Lavoisier, p (3-10, 20-21)*

407.   **Viau C, Tardif R 2003,** Toxicology, In: *Environnement et sante publique - Fondements et pratiques, pp. 119-143. Gerin M, Gosselin P, Cordier S, Viau C, Quenel P, Dewailly E, editors. Edisem / Tec & Doc, Acton Vale / Paris*

408.   **Viguier E and Degorce F. 1992,** Elements anatomiques fondamentaux en chirurgie cutanee plastique et reconstructrice chez les carnivores domestiques, *Point Veterinaire **24**: 5-19*

409.   **Vijaimohan KM, Jainu KE, Sabitha S, Subramaniyam C, Aandhan CS and Shyamala D.2006,** Beneficial effects of alpha linolenic acid rich flaxseed oil on growth performance and hepatic cholesterol metabolism in high fat diet fed rats, *Life Sci **79** (5): 448-454*

410.   **Vogt, A., McElwee, K. J., Blume-Peytavi, U. 2008.**Biology of the hair follicle. In Blume- Peytavi, U., Tosti A., Whiting D., Trueb R. Germany, Springer Verlag. Hair Growth and Disorders. Ref Type: Serial (Book,Monograph)

411.   **Vyas N, Raj Kumar Keservani, Amit Nayak, Sarang Jain, SinghalM. 2010,** Effect of *Tamarindus indica* and *Curcuma longa* on stress induced alopecia *harmacologyonline 1: 377-384*

412.   **Waldron DR and Zimermman P. 2003,** Superficial skin wound in textbook of small animal surgery, *3eme edition. Slatter WB Saunders:258-73*

413.   **Walji R, Boon H, Barnes J, Austin Z, Welsh S and Baker GR.2010,** Consumers of natural health products:natural-born pharmacovigilantes? *BioMedCentral Complementary Alternetive. Medicine **25**:10:8*

414.   **Waltner-Law ME, Wang XL,Law BK, Hall RK, Nawano M and Granner**

DK.2002, Epigallocatechin gallate, a constituent of green tea, represses hepatic glucose production, *Journal of Biological Chemistry 277 : 34933 - 34940*

415. **Wang E and Mcelwee KJ. 2011,** Etiopathogenesis of alopecia areata:Why do our patients get it? *Dermatologic therapy 24:337-347*

416. **Waylan AT, Dunn JD, Johnson BJ, Kayser JP and Sissom EK. 2004,** Effect of flax supplementation and growth promotants on lipoprotein lipase and glycogenin messenger RNA concentrations in finishing cattle, *Journal of Animal Science 82(6): 1868-1875*

417. **Weill P and Mairess G. 2010,** Flax, its oil, its seed, and our health. *Phytotherapie 8: 1-5*

418. **Weill P, Chesneau G, Normand J and Mourot CM.2004,** Qualite lipidique des viandes. Effet du regime ou de l'espece? Quelques observations sur bovins, porcs rabbins et poulets, *Nutrition Clinique et Metabolisme 18:71-75*

419. **Wheater PR, Burkitt HG, Daniels VG, Young B and Heath JW.1995,** Functional Histology, *Third Edition, Arnette Ed: 116-119*

420. **Whiting DA.1993,** Diagnostic and predictive value of horizontal sections of scalp biopsy specimens in male pattern androgenetic alopecia, *J. Am. Acad Dermatol 28: 755-763*

421. **Williams JM.1999,** Open wound management. In FOWLER, D., WILLIAMS, J.M. *BSAVA, Manual of canine and feline wound management and reconstruction, 1st Ed, Cheltenham, BSAVA (British Small Animal Veterinary Association): 37-46. 123-136*

422. **Xu, RX. ,Xiao M. 2003,** The mechanism of Burn Regenerative Therapy and wound healing. The Chinese Journal of Burns Wounds and Surface Ulcers (4): 262-271

423. **Yahya Mahmoudi. 1992,** La therapie par les communes en Algerie. Ain taya edition, P 89

424. **Yamada H, Kiyohara, H. 1999,** Complement-activating polysaccharides from medicinal herbs. In Immunomodulatory agents from plants. H. Wagner, Birkhauser, Basel; 161-202

425. **Yoon Jung IN, Sharif M, Al-Reza, Sun ChUL K. 2010,** Hair growth promoting effect of *zizyphus jujube* Essential oil, *Food and Chemical Toxicology 48*: 1350-1354

426. **Yu M, Finner A, Shapiro J, LO B, Barekatain A and Mcelwee KJ.2006,** Hair follicles and their role in skin health, *Exp. Rev. Dermatol 1*: 855-871

427. **Zanwar Anand A, Aswar Urmila M, Hegde Mahabaleshwar V, Bodhankar Subhash L. 2010,** Estrogenic and Embryo-Fetotoxic Effects of Ethanol Extract of *Linum usitatissimum* in Rats, *Journal of Complementary and Integrative Medicine 7(1): 21*

428. **Zinai D. 2008,** Les brulures, www.blouseblanches.org (accessed 03-032013)

ANNEXES

ANNEX 1: Composition of linseed oil

Compose	Fatty acid family	Content per 100 g
Vitamin K	-	-
Vitamin E	-	17.5 mg
Total saturated fatty acids	-	9,4 g
Total polyunsaturated fatty acids	-	66 g
Total monounsaturated fatty acids	-	20,2 g
Trans fatty acids	-	0,019 g
Erucastic acid (mono-unsaturated)	w-9	0,13 g
Stearic acid (saturated)	-	3,428 g
Pentadecanoic acid (saturated)	-	0,014 g
Palmitoleic acid (monounsaturated)	w-7	0,046 g
Palmitic acid (saturated)	-	6,047 g
Oleic acid (monounsaturated)	w-9	18,115 g
Myristic acid (saturated)	-	0,041 g
Linoleic acid (polyunsaturated)	w-6	15,553 g
Lignoceric acid (saturated)	-	0,078 g
Heptadecanoic acid (saturated)	-	0,046 g
Cetoleic acid (monounsaturated)	w-11	0,068 g
Behenic acid (saturated)	-	0,068 g
Arachidic acid (saturated)	-	0,146 g
Alpha-linolenic acid (polyunsaturated)	w-3	56,018 g

The fatty acid composition of the **triglycerides** in linseed oil is as follows:

- a-linolenic acid: 45 - 70
- linoleic acid: 12 - 24%.
- oleic acid: 10 - 21 %.
- saturated fatty acids: 6 - 18

The nutritional analysis, for 5 mL of a typical food flaxseed oil, is as follows:

Energy	Protein (g)	Fat (g)	Carbohydrates (g)
42 Cal	0	4,7	0
176 KJ		Of which fatty acids: • satures: 0.4 g • monoinsatures: 0.8 g • polyunsaturated: 3.5 g • linoleic: 0.6 g	

(Source: Souci, Fachmann, Kraut: The composition of foods. Tables of nutritional values, 7th edition, 2008, MedPharm Scientific Publishers / Taylor & Francis).

Energy input		Main components		Minerals & Oligo-elements (mg)		Vitamins (mg)		Fatty acids (mg)	
Joules (KJ)	1558	Carbohydrates O g -		calcium	198	Vit B1	0,170	Palmitic acid	1840
(calories)(Kcal)	376	Starch O g - Sugars O g		Chrome	0,00581	Vit B2	0,160	Stearic acid	1110
				cobalt	0,0056	Vit B3 (or PP)	1,4	Oleic acid	5620
		Dietary fibres	38,6 g	copper	1,2	Vit K	0,005	Linoleic acid	4200
		Protein	24,4 g	Iron	8,2			Alpha linolenic acid	16700
		Fat 30.9 g — Satures 2950 mg		Manganese	2,6				
				Nickel	0,190				
		— omega- 3 16700 mg		Phosphorus	662				
				Potassium	725				
		— omega -6 4200 mg		Sodium	607				
		— omega-9 5620 mg							
		Water	6,10 g	Zinc	5.5 mg				

ANNEX 3: Composition of the products tested

Product	Origin	Composition
Linseed oil (HUL)	Dr Abdenour,	

		Allantoin , Guaiazulene , Active ingredientsParachlorometacresol , Alpha tocopherol (E307)
Cicatryl-Bio® (CIC)	Private Pharmacy	Methyl parahydroxybenzoate (E218), Propyl parahydroxybenzoate (E216), Paraffin, Vaseline, Glycerol monostearate, Macrogol, . $_x$ Sorbitol (E420), Purified water, Excipients Mixture of : Cetostearic alcohol, Sodium cetyl stearyl sulfate, Mixture of : Cetostearyl alcohol, Sodium cetyl stearyl sulfate, Ethoxyl fatty acid
Vaseline (VAS)		

APPENDIX 4: Material for the study of epithelial regeneration

- Shaving equipment
-Mower
-Razor blade
-Aluminium foil.
• **Anesthesia products**
-Ketamine hydrochloride (diazepam)
-Xylocaine (Lidocaine)
• **Burns material**
-Masselotte
-Boiling water
• **Products tested**
-The essential oil is provided by the herbalist Abdenour (Abdenour, 2008)
-Cicatryl-Bio ® (Appendix 4) and Vaseline are purchased from a pharmacist.
- Measuring equipment
-    Ordinary scale (NEW CROWN, D: 0.01, Max: 30Kg)
-    Electronic caliper (0.001 mm accuracy)
-    Pencil and transparent paper
- Tissue collection equipment
-Anatomical dissection kit
-10% formaldehyde pills
- Histology equipment
-Note block: macroscopy information
-Solvent: paraffin alcohol, xylene, water
-Dye: hematoxylin, eosin.
-Consumables

ANNEX 5: Consumables

• Markers
• Ink and pencils
• Coplin bottle for colouring
• Slide rack for staining and drying
• Blades
• Slats
• Pliers
• Mounting medium such as Permount

APPENDIX 6: Rabbit Individual Information Sheet

Arrival	Origin	Cage number	Rabbit number	Age	Report	Background	Treatment

Weekly weighing

JO	J7	J15	J21	J28
Weight				
observation				

APPENDIX 7: Tissue treatment programme

Bac number	Solvent	Time	Observation
1	80° alcohol	45 minutes	Before placing the basket containing the cassettes in the 1er tray, it must be well drained
2	90° alcohol	45 minutes	Drain before moving on to the next bin
3	100° alcohol	45 minutes	Drain before moving on to the next bin
4	100° alcohol	45 minutes	Drain before moving on to the next bin
5	100° alcohol	45 minutes	Drain before moving on to the next bin
6	100° alcohol	1 hour	Drain before moving on to the next bin
7	100° alcohol	1 hour	Drain very well before putting in the xylene tank
8	Xylene	45 minutes	Drain before moving on to the next bin
9	Xylene	45 minutes	Drain before moving on to the next bin
10	Xylene	45 minutes	Drain very well before putting in the paraffin tray
11	Paraffin	2 hours	Tapes can be left overnight in paraffin

APPENDIX 8: Standard Hemalun Eosin Stain

Bac number	Solvent	Time	Observation
1	Xylene	15 mnts	
2	Xylene	15 mnts	
3	90° alcohol	1 mnt	
4	100° alcohol	1 mnt	
5	100° alcohol	1 mnt	
6	Water (H$_2$O)		Until the tissue is bleached
7	Hemalun		(Haris Hematoxylin) rapid passage when the solution is new
8	Water	1 mnt	Wash well, so as not to mix the dyes
9	Eosin	3-20 mints	Enriching the solvent; the more it ages, the longer it takes
10	Water	Washing	Washing well to keep the alcohol tray clean
11	100° alcohol	Passage	
12	Xylene	Passage	
13	Xylene	Passage	
14	Xylene	Passage	
15	Xylene		Up to 1mnt
16	Assembly		Cover with a coverslip using mounting fluid (Eukit)

- Plant material
-    Linseed oil
-    Vaseline oil
-    Ground flaxseed.
•   **Shaving equipment**
-Tape measure
-Marker
-Mower
-Aluminium foil.
•   **Measuring equipment**
-Graduated rule
-Micrometer (figure)
-Microscope
-Precision balance (KERN plus, Max=510, d=0,001g)
- Animal material
-Rabbit (page 57)
- Observation equipment
-Information sheet
-Ordinary scale (Max=30kg)
- Blood sampling equipment
-Cotton and alcohol
-Heparin needles and tubes vacutainer
-Centrifuge (Hettich zentrifugen EBA 20)
- Biochemical analysis equipment
-PLC (C1 8200 Architect)
-Kits
- Histology and tissue sampling equipment
Idem (page 58)
APPENDIX 11: Material for the zootechnical performance study
- Animal material
-Rabbits (page 57)
•   **Weighing equipment**
-Ordinary scale
•   **Felling equipment**
-Dissecting kit
-Precision scale
•   **Calculation equipment**
-Data from the individual sheets transferred to Excel.
-Matlab v7.7.0.2162 (Release 2008b)

Latin name	Common Name	Name Arab
Abrus Precatorius L	Jequirity, crab eye, rosary bean Wild licorice.	
Ageratum Conyzoides	**Whiteweed** Chickweed Goatweed	
Aloe Barbadensis	Aloe vera or Aloes.	
Allium Sativum	Garlic.	
Asiasari Radix	Wild Chinese ginger root.	
Butea monosperma	Flame of the f o re t, kino bengal .	
Cassia fistula	Golden Rain Tree	
Cedrus Atlantica	Atlas Cedar	
Centella asiatica	Centella and Gotu Kola	
Cinnamomum zeylanicum	Ceylon cinnamon.	
Cocos nucifera.	The Coconut Palm.	
Copaifera langsdorffii oleoresin	Copahier, Balsam of Copahu, Balsam of Copahu	
Datura alba	Datura Metel	
Eclipta alba	false daisy" false daisy	
Embelia ribes	False Black Pepper, White-flowered Embelia: White flowered	
Fagopyrum Esculentum	Ble noir	
Glycyrrhiza Glabra	Glabrous Reglisse	
Hibiscus Rosa Sinensis Linn	Hibiscus rose de Chine, Hibiscus de Chine, Rose de Chine, Rose de Cayenne.	
Napoleons Imperialis	Napoleons Hat :Napolaon Hat	
Inula Viscosa	False yellowhead :False yellow Tate ; Slimy inula.	
Juneperus Oxycedrus,	Genavrier oxycadre, Oxycadre, Arbre a Cade, Cade, Petit Cade d'Espagne.	
Kniphofia uvalaria Moench	Tritoma, red hot poker, lily torch.	
Lawsonia Inermis	Henna	
Ocimum Gratissimum	African Basil, Big Balm, Mint Gabonese,Tolsi,Basil tree	
Opilia Celtidifolia	"konon-gbai": gbai of birds.	
Opuntia ficus indica	Prickly pear, prickly pear cactus	
Pinus Halepensis	Aleppo pine, Jerusalem pine, white pine	
Prunus Dulcis	Almond tree.	
Pterocarpus Angolensis	Kiaat tree, Mokwa, Moroto, wild teak.	
Pterocarpus santalinus	"Red sandalwood	
Rubus Sanctusa.	Rubus:Bramble Sanctus:Sacra , Blackberry: ripe ,	
Russelia Equisetiformis	patard plant , Coral plant ,Coral fountain , Coralblow and usinede Fountain .	
Sphaeranthus Indicus	East Indian dumplings, Mundi	
Teucrium Polium	Germandrae tomenteuse Germandrae greyish-white	
Tephrosia purpurea	Indigo-red, the purple taphrosia	
erminilia chebula		
Tragic involucrata		
Trichosanthes Dioica	Pointed flask	
Zizyphus Jujuba	Jujubier, red date or black date.	
Zizyphus Oenoplia	Jackal Jujube :Chacal Jujubeir, Small-fruited Jujube :small fruits of jujube or Wild Jujube.	